MW01485880

Questions and Answers

2nd Edition

Volume 1

By Stu Silverstein, M.D., FAAP

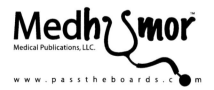

Medhumor
Medical Publications, LLC.

www.passtheboards.com

MedHumor Medical Publications, Stamford, Connecticut

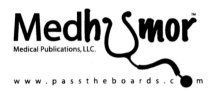

www.passtheboards.com

Published by:
Medhumor Medical Publications, LLC
1127 High Ridge Road, Suite 332
Stamford, CT 06905 U.S.A.

ISBN: **0-9771374-8-1**

First Edition Copyright © 2000 Medhumor Medical Publications, LLC
Second Edition Copyright © 2008 Medhumor Medical Publications, LLC

Printed in the United States of America

This book is designed to provide information and guidance in regard to the subject matter covered. It is to be used as a study guide for physicians preparing for the General Pediatric Certifying Exam administered by the American Board of Pediatrics. It is not meant to be a clinical manual. The reader is advised to consult textbooks and other reference manuals in making clinical decisions. It is not the purpose of this book to reprint all the information that is otherwise available, but rather to assist the Board Candidate in organizing the material to facilitate study and recall on the exam. The reader is encouraged to read other sources of material, in particular picture atlases that are available.

Although every precaution has been taken in the preparation of this book, the publisher, author, and members of the editorial board assume no responsibility for errors, omissions or typographical mistakes. Neither is any liability assumed for damages resulting from the direct and indirect use of the information contained herein. The book contains information that is up-to-date only up to the printing date. Due to the very nature of the medical profession, there will be points out-of-date as soon as the book rolls off the press. The purpose of this book is to educate and entertain.

**If you do not wish to be bound by the above,
you may return this book to the publisher for a full refund.**

Publisher:	MedHumor Medical Publications, LLC Stamford, CT
VP/Content Development :	Stuart Silverstein, MD, FAAP Clinical Director Firefly After Hours Pediatrics, LLC Stamford, CT Assistant Clinical Professor Emergency Medicine New York Medical College
Senior Editor:	Jon Durica, MD Stamford, CT
General Manager/ Operations:	Todd Van Allen
Design / Copy Editor:	Antoinette D'Amore, A.D. Design www.addesign-graphics.com
Cover Designer:	Rachel Mindrup www.rmindrup.com

About the Author

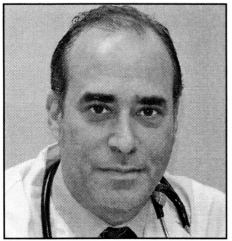

Dr. Stu Silverstein is the founder and CEO of Medhumor Medical Publications, LLC which began with the publication of the critically acclaimed "Laughing your way to Passing the Pediatric Boards"™ back in the spring of 2000. Word spread quickly that finally there was a book out there that turned a traditionally daunting process into one that was actually fun and enjoyable. This groundbreaking study guide truly "Took the Boredom out of Board review"® with reports from our readers that they were able to reduce their study and review time in half. Those who were taking the exam for the 2nd time not only passed but increased their scores dramatically.

Their supplementary pediatric titles have also been crtically acclaimed. Medhumor Publications LLC, has since expanded their catalogue to include a title for the USMLE Step 3 and the Neurolgy Board exams.

The concept of the "Laughing your way to Passing the Boards"™ and Medhumor Medical Publications, LLC were conceived by Dr. Silverstein. He brought his years of experience in the field of Standup Comedy and Comedy writing after he realized the critical need for a study guide that spoke the language of colleagues rather than the language of dusty textbooks. His work as a Standup Comedian and Medical Humorist has frequently been featured in several newspapers, radio programs and TV shows, including the New York Times, WCBS newsradio in NY City, as well as World News Tonight with Peter Jennings.

Dr. Silverstein has also served as a contributing editor for the <u>Resident and Staff Physician</u> annual board review issue and has authored numerous articles on medical humor. He has served on the faculty of the Osler Institute Board Review course, UCLA Pediatric Board Review course and several local board review courses. He is the co-author of "What about Me? Growing up with a Developmentally Disabled Sibling" written with Dr. Bryna Siegel, professor of Child Psychiatry , the University of California San Francisco. Dr. Silverstein is in demand as a lecturer for residency programs on successful preparation for the pediatric board exam.

In addition to writing, lecturing, and expanding the scope of Medhumor Medical Publications, LLC., Dr. Silverstein is the Clinical Director for Firefly After Hours Pediatrics, a subacute emergency practice. Dr. Silverstein is an Assistant Clinical Professor of Emergency Medicine at the New York Medical College in Valhalla, New York.

Questions and Answers Volume 1 (2nd Edition)

In putting together the 2nd edition of our *Question and Answer* series we did our utmost to incorporate the suggestions of our readers who successfully passed the General Pediatric Board Exam as well as the Recertification Exam.

Each book now contains 400 questions each broken down by subspecialty. This allows the reader to focus on areas that need improvement. Matching and questions based on clinical vignettes now count as one question. Therefore the 2nd edition contains significantly more questions than the 1st editions.

All questions have been reviewed and revised based on the content specifications published by the American Academy of Pediatrics. The infectious disease and preventive medicine questions were updated based on the most up to date information published in the online edition of the AAP "Red Book".

We hope that these updated *Question and Answer* books will continue to serve those for whom passing the pediatric certification and recertification exams is the next ticket to be punched.

—Stuart Silverstein, MD, FAAP
Stamford, CT

Table of Contents

Answers **141**

Icon Signposts

The answer sections contain several icon signposts indicating the significance of the highlighted material as follows:

BUZZ WORDS	*Buzz Words*	This describes buzzwords or key phrases that are typical for a given disorder. By learning this, you will often be able to recognize the answer in the wording of the question itself.
EITHER OR CHOICES	*Down to two choices*	This points out minute differences between similar disorders, which are critical to answering many questions correctly.

Questions

Adolescent

1)   A 13 year old boy in your practice shouts, "NO!" when you ask if he has any questions prior to your doing a routine physical. His mother, in a shrill voice that actually DOES peel the paint off all 4 walls, says, "Go ahead, and ask him. He's a doctor." The patient meekly says, "Doc, I've got one breast that is actually bigger than those of some of the girls in my class. What's the deal?" Fortunately, you are wearing a bow-tie that day and you deliver the following in your most professorial tone:

A)   This is quite rare among *non*-marijuana users
B)   It is due to estrogen excess that is short lived, and he will outgrow it
C)   It will resolve once he is producing adequate testosterone
D)   It occurs in 75% of adolescent boys
E)   It will spontaneously resolve without intervention in virtually all cases
F)   Ask if he interested in purchasing the "bro" or as it is sometimes known the "male bra" [1]

2)   The parents of a 13-year-old girl are concerned about her pubertal development. On physical exam you note moderate breast development, with glandular tissue beyond the areolae. However, you confirm that there is no secondary mounding of the nipples or areolae. Which of the following is the most appropriate sex maturity rating for breast development for this patient?

A)   1
B)   2
C)   3
D)   4
E)   5

---

[1] Yes this is not original we saw it on an episode of "Seinfeld" too.

3)   A 12-year-old, premenarchal girl presents with intermittent white vaginal discharge over the past 2 to 3 months. She is Tanner stage 2 on physical exam, and the rest of the physical exam is normal. Vaginal smear reveals 2 leukocytes/HPF as well as superficial vaginal cells. Which of the following is the MOST appropriate management?

A) Metronidazole vaginal suppository vaginal culture for Chlamydia trachomatis
B) Vaginal culture for Gardnerella vaginalis
C) Immediate referral to child protective services after obtaining appropriate cultures
D) Reassurance that the discharge is normal

4)   A 17-year-old football player has been fatigued since the conclusion of the football season one week ago. Prior to that time he had been doing well.

During the last game of the season he was hit in the left thigh during a tackle but he toughed it out and continued to play. On physical exam he still has pain and is walking with a limp. His white blood cell count is 10.0. His HCT is now 35, and at last year's physical examination he had an HCT of 42. His ESR is 6 and his electrolytes are all within normal limits and he has a serum alkaline phosphatase level of 200 and lactic dehydrogenase of 225. The MOST likely diagnosis is:

A) Osteoid osteoma
B) Osteogenic sarcoma
C) Osteomyelitis
D) Deep thigh hematoma
E) Anabolic steroid use

5)   You are asked to give a lecture to a group of high school coaches who want to know how to prevent "heat-related illnesses". Which of the following is the most appropriate recommendation?

A) Table salt tablets daily
B) Wear clothing that is loose fitting, light colored yet tasteful and not "Tutee Fruity"
C) Acclimatize the athletes over 5 days when training in the summer
D) Practice at night.
E) Provide unrestricted access to fluids

6)	Each of the following is true regarding Chlamydia infection in adolescent females EXCEPT

   A)	Sterile pyuria is common
   B)	70% of endocervical infections are asymptomatic
   C)	Diagnosis based solely on physical examination is unreliable
   D)	Perihepatitis and endometriosis are possible complications
   E)	Hepatitis and endometriosis are possible complications

7)	Last month you evaluated an 18 year old male and prescribed 1 Gram single dose of azithromycin for a documented Chlamydia infection. He confirms that he has had only "one sexual partner" who he brings with him this time to be tested. He now presents with a one week history of urethritis with discharge confirmed on physical exam. Culture confirms that he once again has chlamydia urethritis. The most likely explanation for the recurrent infection is:

   A)	He has more than one sexual partner
   B)	Poor compliance
   C)	Reinfection with his untreated partner
   D)	He also has gonococcal urethritis
   E)	He needs a broader spectrum antibiotic

8)	The ideal body weight in females can be calculated as follows:

   A)	50 pounds for 50 inches in height plus 2 pounds for each additional inch
   B)	75 pounds for 75 inches in height plus 5 pounds for each additional inch
   C)	100 pounds for 60 inches in height plus 5 pounds for each additional inch
   D)	125 pounds for every 72 inches of height plus 10 pounds for each additional inch
   E)	125 pounds for every 72 inches of height plus 5 pounds for each additional inch

9) With regards to anorexia nervosa: Each of the following in an otherwise clinically stable patient would be an indication for hospital admission EXCEPT for:

A) Heart rate greater than 100
B) Heart rate less than 40
C) Systolic blood pressure less than 90 mm Hg
D) Prolonged QT interval on EKG

10) You are evaluating a 16 year old female presenting with dysfunctional uterine bleeding. Her menstrual cycles last 6 days and occur every 19 days. Her hemoglobin is 11 and her vital signs are stable. Each of the following would be appropriate treatment at this time *except* for:

A) Oral contraceptive pills
B) Serial hematocrits
C) Hospital admission for packed red cell transfusion
D) Iron supplements
E) Maintain a menstrual calendar

Allergy & Immunology

11) Match the disorders on the left with underlying etiology on the right.

1) Severe combined immunodeficiency
2) Bruton's disease
3) Common variable immunodeficiency
4) Di George syndrome
5) HIV
6) The "Bubble Boy" in *Seinfeld*

(A) Primarily affects B cells
(B) T and B cell counts are normal
(C) Adenosine deaminase deficiency
(D) Associated with hypocalcemia
(E) Elevated immunoglobulins
(F) Elevated T cells

12) Meningococcemia is most likely to be seen in a patient with which one of the following disorders?

A) X-linked agammaglobulinemia
B) IgA deficiency
C) DiGeorge syndrome
D) Ataxia-telangiectasia
E) Complement deficiency

13) A patient with deficiency of C6 would be MOST at risk for infection with which of the following infectious agents?

A) *Staph aureus*
B) *Neisseria meningococcus*
C) *Neisseria gonococcus*
D) Group B *Strep*
E) *Neisseria meningococcus* and *Neisseria gonococcus*

14) A 6-month-old infant presents with recurrent vomiting and diarrhea. On physical examination, the infant appears to be pale and somewhat cyanotic. The infant was fed standard formula several hours ago; otherwise, the history is unremarkable. Which of the following statements is MOST accurate regarding the infant's condition?

A) Skin testing with cow milk allergen would be indicated.
B) The symptoms are likely to be cardiac in origin.
C) The symptoms are likely due to a TE fistula.
D) It is most likely non-IgE hypersensitivity reaction to the formula.
E) It is most likely an IgE-mediated reaction to the formula.

15) A 2-year-old boy with eczema has had recurrent respiratory infections, including *Pneumocystis carinii* pneumonia. Lab studies show thrombocytopenia and normal serum immunoglobulin concentrations. Which of the following is the most likely diagnosis?

A) Chronic granulomatous disease
B) AIDS
C) DiGeorge syndrome
D) Thrombotic thrombocytopenia
E) Wiskott-Aldrich syndrome

16) You are asked to consult on an 18 month old toddler with more than 10 episodes of otitis media and 2 hospitalizations for lobar pneumonia. His past history is significant for frequent bruising and chronic eczema. The most likely diagnosis is:

A) Chronic myelogenous leukemia
B) Kartagener's syndrome
C) Job syndrome
D) Wiskott-Aldrich Syndrome
E) DiGeorge syndrome

17) Each of the following is true regarding ataxia telangiectasia *except*

A) Autosomal dominant
B) Presents in early childhood with regression of motor milestones
C) Recurrent sinopulmonary infections
D) Depressed IgA levels
E) Increased risk of malignancy

18)   **Each of the following is true regarding chronic granulomatous disease** *except:*

A) All forms are inherited in an X-liked recessive pattern
B) It can be diagnosed with the *dihydrorhodamine flow cytometry test*
C) Bowel obstruction is a complication
D) Prophylactic treatment with trimethoprim/sulfamethoxazole is indicated
E) Prophylaxis treatment with itraconazole is indicated

19)   **Which of the following medications can be expected to** *reduce* **theophylline levels in the blood?**

A) Cimetidine
B) Ranitidine
C) Rifampin
D) Phenobarbital
E) C and D

20)   **Which of the following is true regarding anaphylactic reactions?**

A) Acute anaphylactic reactions can be treated with oral diphenhydramine
B) Acute anaphylactic reactions can be treated with oral corticosteroids
C) Acute anaphylactic reactions should be treated with 0.01 mg/kg of epinephrine (1:10,000) SQ
D) Acute anaphylactic reactions should be treated with 0.01 mg/kg of epinephrine (1:1000) SQ
E) Acute anaphylactic reactions should be treated with 0.1 mg/kg of epinephrine (1:1000) SQ

Cardiology

21) **Each of the following is common non-cardiac causes of chest pain EXCEPT:**

A) Costochondritis
B) Anxiety
C) Exercise-induced asthma
D) Foreign body aspiration
E) Pleural effusion

22) **Match the EKG finding on the left with the diagnosis on the right.**

1) Left ventricular hypertrophy   (A) AV canal defect
2) Right axis deviation   (B) Tetralogy of Fallot
3) Left axis deviation   (C) Aortic stenosis

23) **Match the innocent murmur on the left with the description on the right.**

1) Still's murmur   (A) Systolic ejection-type murmur heard best over the upper left sternal border
2) Pulmonary flow murmur   (B) Low in pitch and often musical in quality
3) Cervical venous hum   (C) Often present only when sitting or standing

24) **An infant diagnosed with tetralogy of Fallot experiences a "hypercyanotic crisis". Which one of the following medications would be *most appropriately* included in the management of this crisis?**

A) Subcutaneous morphine
B) Intramuscular phenobarbital
C) Oral Xanax® (alprazolam)
D) A trip to the Vulcan city of Xanadu
E) Intravenous calcium

25) **A 4-year-old child has been on digoxin for over one year. He presents in the ER with headache, fatigue, and muscle weakness. He is also experiencing a loss of appetite. The MOST appropriate next step would be to:**

A) Obtain CBC, electrolyte levels; administer 20cc/kg Normal Saline and discharge to cardiology
B) Obtain digoxin level and admit for observation
C) Obtain digoxin level, EKG, chest x-ray; if within normal limits, discharge after a period of observation
D) Hold digoxin, decrease digoxin dose, and obtain dig level in one day
E) Hold digoxin, decrease digoxin dose, and obtain dig level in one week

26) **A 7-year-old born with tricuspid atresia is sent to you because she is complaining of severe headaches coupled with vomiting for the past 3 days. She is afebrile and somewhat lethargic. Her physical examination her hematocrit is 53 and her WBC and the remainder of her labs are all normal. Which of the following is the MOST appropriate next diagnostic step?**

A) Examination of CSF
B) Restriction of intake to clear fluids reexamination in 24 hours
C) X-ray study of the skull
D) Brain scan using technetium
E) Head CT

27) The parents of an asymptomatic 7-year-old boy with small VSD ask for your opinion regarding his participation in sports-related activities. Which of the following would be the MOST appropriate advice?

A) If activity is not partially restricted, he is at risk for the development of pulmonary hypertension
B) Sustained isometric exercise should be avoided
C) Competitive track running is associated with an increased incidence of syncope
D) He can participate in all sports without risks
E) Activity should be restricted in high school, but limitations are unnecessary at this time

28) Which of the following drugs is MOST likely to be effective in *decreasing cardiac afterload* by decreasing systemic resistance?

A) Digoxin
B) Furosemide
C) Spironolactone
D) Chlorothiazide
E) Captopril

29) Syncope in a teenager brought on by which of the following is most ominous?

A) Defecation
B) Exercise
C) Headache
D) Seizure
E) Standing still and urinating

30) **The Cardiac cath oxygen saturation and pressure gradient demonstrated below is most consistent with:**

A) Normal Heart
B) Tetralogy of Fallot
C) Total Anomalous venous return
D) Pulmonary stenosis
E) Aortic stenosis

	(SVC)	70%		95%		(PV)

	2	5
(RA)		(LA)
	70%	95%

	22/2	110/10
(RV)		(LV)
	70%	95%

PA	30/15	110/70	A
	70%	95%	

31)   The Cardiac cath oxygen saturation and pressure gradient demonstrated below is most consistent with:

A) Normal heart
B) Tetralogy of Fallot
C) Truncus arteriosis
D) Total anomalous venous return
E) Transposition of the great vessels

(SVC)	70%		95%	(PV)
(RA)	2		5	(LA)
	70%		95%	
(RV)	110/70		50/5	(LV)
	70%		95%	
PA	110/70		50/5	A
	70%		95%	

32) **The Cardiac cath oxygen saturation and pressure gradient demonstrated below is most consistent with**

A) Normal heart
B) Tetralogy of Fallot
C) Pulmonary stenosis
D) Aortic stenosis
E) Transposition of the great vessels

(SVC)	70%		95%		(PV)
(RA)	2		5		(LA)
	70%		95%		
(RV)	25/5		110/10		(LV)
	70%		95%		
PA	1		110/70		A
	70%		95%		

33) **The Cardiac cath oxygen saturation and pressure gradient demonstrated below is most consistent with:**

A) Pulmonary stenosis
B) ASD
C) VSD
D) Aortic stenosis
E) Transposition of the great vessels

(SVC)	70%		95%		(PV)
(RA)	2		5		(LA)
	70%		95%		
(RV)	30/4		110/10		(LV)
	85%		95%		
PA	30/15		110/70		A
	85%		95%		

34) **The Cardiac cath oxygen saturation and pressure gradient demonstrated below is most consistent with:**

A) Normal heart
B) Tetralogy of Fallot
C) Total anomalous venous return
D) Pulmonary stenosis
E) Aortic stenosis

(SVC)	70%	95%	(PV)
(RA)	2 / 70%	5 / 95%	(LA)
(RV)	22/2 / 70%	120/18 / 95%	(LV)
PA	30/15 / 70%	80/50 / 95%	A

35) You are evaluating a 16 year old high school varsity athlete whose 45 year old father is being treated for "high triglycerides or something like that" says the 16 year old.

Recently he has been experiencing chest pain which radiates to the left shoulder which feels like pressure. On physical exam there is no abdominal pain, no chest pain with palpation. His blood pressure is 110/72 with no heart murmur noted.

The most appropriate step in managing this patient would be:

A) Trial of antacids no restrictions on playing ball
B) Abdominal CT with IV contrast to assess for cholecystitis
C) Trial of ibuprofen and no restrictions
D) EKG if not ST changes clear for full activity
E) Cardiology referral and restriction of sports and other strenuous exercise

36) Each of the following are seen in both simple atrioseptal defect and total anomalous venous return *except* for:

A) Palpable sternal lift
B) Tachypnea
C) Fixed splitting of S2
D) Cyanosis
E) Pulmonary flow murmur

Cognition, Language & Learning

37) A child at what age can expect a stranger to understand 75% of what he says?

A) 24 months old
B) 36 months old
C) 18 months old
D) 18 years old
E) Presidential candidate

38) **Identifying those children who are at highest risk for, or who have developmental disabilities, is best achieved by:**

A) EEG monitoring while watching the auditions for American Idol
B) Screening all high-risk infants for hearing loss
C) The Denver Developmental and vision screen
D) Screening all children for vision, hearing and language deficits
E) Screening for inborn errors of metabolism at birth

39) **A 14 year old male with mild retardation presents with a past medical history that is unremarkable. The family history is essentially positive for a couple of uncles who, according to the mother, "are 5 beers short of a 6-pack" and according to the father, "were one top short of the 4 tops".**

On physical exam you note a long face that would rival Richard Belzer on Law and Order, large ears and macroorchidism. This disorder would *BEST* be diagnosed with which study?

A) Head CT
B) Head MRI
C) Karyotype
D) EEG
E) BBC

40) **Eligibility for medicaid and social security benefits for children with mental retardation is dependent on:**

A) They become eligible at age 18 regardless of parents ability to provide for the child
B) They become eligible at age 18 if the parents lack the financial means to provide for the child
C) They become eligible at age 21 regardless of parents ability to provide for the child
D) They become eligible at age 21 if the parents lack the financial means to provide for the child
E) They are eligible as soon as they are diagnosed

41) The key element in *"Individual Education Plans"* (IEP) for children with *severe* mental retardation is:

A) Anticonvulsants to treat irritability and mood swings
B) Anticonvulsants to control seizures
C) Alpha-2-adrenergic agents to control aggression and self-injurious behaviors
D) Behavioral management strategies
E) Tutoring and vocational training

Critical Care

42) You are on call 5th night on call in the PICU in 4 days. You need to start a child on a ventilator, and you need to quickly calculate the tidal volume for this 15kg child. The tidal volume is closest to:

A) 1500 ml
B) 150 ml
C) 100 ml
D) 60 ml
E) 35 ml
F) 6 trillion ml

43) This month you are working in the PICU and you are successfully managing a case with a routine case of botulism poisoning. You are there catching up on your dictation, noting the steady drone of the Mom's clicking on her laptop when she stops, your eyes meet and she says, "So Doc, what exactly is the mechanism of action of botulism toxin?"

You've done your homework and correctly answer her with:

A) It increases reuptake of acetylcholine at the presynaptic neuron
B) It blocks the mom's laptop from "googling" botulism toxin
C) It destroys the postsynaptic membrane
D) It blocks release of acetylcholine from the presynaptic neuron
E) It blocks the reuptake of acetylcholine

44) **You arrive at a swimming pool just as lifeguards are rescuing a toddler from the swimming pool. The toddler is limp, and appears to be unconscious and making minimal respiratory efforts. The best immediate intervention would be:**

A) The Heimlich maneuver to clear the airway of water
B) Turn the child on the side in the prone position followed by 3 back blows
C) Place the child on his back and lift his left leg up and down pumping aspirated water out of his mouth, like in Tom and Jerry and other cartoons
D) Initiate BLS including rescue breathing and chest compressions if indicated
E) Immobilize cervical spine and call 911

45) **Which of the following is the *diagnostic triad* of Adult Respiratory Distress Syndrome (ARDS)?**

A) Cardiogenic pulmonary edema, impaired oxygenation, bilateral pulmonary infiltrates
B) Noncardiogenic pulmonary edema, impaired oxygenation, bilateral pulmonary infiltrates
C) Renal failure, impaired oxygenation, unilateral pulmonary infiltrates
D) Renal failure, impaired oxygenation, bilateral pulmonary infiltrates
E) Noncardiogenic pulmonary edema, acidosis, bilateral pulmonary infiltrates

46) **Which of the following is pathognomic for brain death?**

A) Complete absence of brainstem function for more than 12 hours for unknown reasons
B) Flat line EEG confirmed by 2 neurologists
C) Irreversible cause with complete absence of brainstem function for 6 hours
D) No blood flow to intracranial arteries confirmed with cerebral nucleotide study
E) The sensation you will feel the day after taking the board exam.

Dermatology

47) **The cutaneous manifestation seen in rheumatic fever is:**

A) Erythema multiforme
B) Erythema marginatum
C) Erythema nodosum
D) Erythema migrans
E) Erythema infectiosum

48) **A 15-month-old girl in your practice has a port-wine stain covering a large portion of her right cheek. The parents are concerned about the appearance and would like to know about treatment options. Which of the following therapies would be the MOST effective and the safest?**

A) Cryotherapy
B) Dermablend®
C) Electrocautery
D) Pulsed dye laser
E) Excision and grafting
F) Contralateral tattooing

49) **In the following set of questions, for each numbered word or phrase, choose the lettered heading that is MOST CLOSELY ASSOCIATED with it. Lettered headings may be selected once, more than once, or not at all.**

1) Primarily involves mucous membranes
2) Parvovirus B19
3) Rash seen in 70% of cases of Lyme disease
4) Associated with inflammatory bowel disease
5) Eyes glazed over trying to determine which erythema is correct on the Exam-ema
6) Erythematous macules on the back

(A) Erythema marginatum
(B) Erythema nodosum
(C) Erythema infectiosum
(D) Erythema multiforme
(E) Erythema migrans
(F) Erythema confusiosum

50)   **Which of the following dermatological manifestations is seen with tuberculosis?**

A)   Erythema confusiosum
B)   Erythema multiforme
C)   Erythema nodosum
D)   Erythema migrans
E)   Erythema infectiosum

51)   **Which of the following lesions is *most consistently* found on children with tuberous sclerosis?**

A)   Cafe au lait spot
B)   Hematomas
C)   Sclerosing tubers
D)   Port wine stains
E)   Ash leaf macules
F)   Periungual fibromas

52)   ***Borrelia burgdorferi* is associated with:**

A)   An extra actor in the movie Goodfellas
B)   Erythema multiforme
C)   Erythema multi-informant
D)   Erythema migrans
E)   Erythema marginatum
F)   Rocky mountain spotted fever

53) A 6-week-old infant presents with a progressively worsening rash. The rash is observed in the axilla, neck, and the diaper area and appears to be yellowish, greasy, and scaly, but non-pruritic. The mother is very concerned; all attempts to treat with "previously prescribed creams" and lotions have not helped. The MOST appropriate next step in managing this infant and the mother's concerns would be:

A) Reassurance
B) Zinc supplements
C) Hydrocortisone cream and nystatin ointment
D) Moisturizing lotions and soap
E) Skin biopsy

54) A 3-month-old former 32-week premie presents with crusty plaques around the mouth and on the face. The plaques have distinct margins. In addition, the infant is irritable and has patches of missing hair and moderate diarrhea. The BEST step in managing this patient would be:

A) Reassurance
B) Zinc supplements
C) Hydrocortisone cream and nystatin ointment
D) Moisturizing lotions and soap
E) Skin biopsy

55) Match the lettered diagnosis on the right with the description on the left.

1) Inflammation and black dots	(A) Alopecia totalis
2) Complete areas of smooth hair loss	(B) Alopecia areata
3) Incomplete patches of hair loss	(C) Tinea capitis
4) Eyebrows are typically involved	(D) Alopecia neurotica
5) Pediatrician preparing for the boards	(E) Trichotillomania

56) A 4-year-old girl is being seen for "infected mosquito bites" on the lower part of her leg. She is also noted to have "puffy" eyelids. With the exception of the crusted lesions on both legs and periorbital edema, her physical exam is normal. Which of the following would be the most appropriate next step?

A) Culture of the material scraped from the skin lesions
B) CBC and ESR
C) Urinalysis
D) Prescription of Pen VK and reexamination in one week
E) Hospitalization

57) A 15-year-old girl has a one-week history of pruritic rash on her back and chest. The rash started with one "spot" approximately 2 cm in size on her chest. She is taking no medication and has no other significant medical history. Physical examination reveals an afebrile patient with a diffuse, hyperpigmented, papular rash on her back and chest. Which of the following is the most likely diagnosis?

A) Pityriasis rosea
B) Psoriasis
C) Keratosis pilaris
D) Lyme disease
E) Parvovirus infection

58) Each of the following conditions is associated with the production of an exotoxin EXCEPT:

A) Scarlet fever
B) Hemolytic uremic syndrome
C) Toxic shock syndrome
D) Toxic epidermal necrolysis
E) Staphylococcal scalded skin syndrome

59) A 13-month-old has an excoriated rash about the neck, wrists, ankles, and genitalia. His mother has a similar pruritic rash. Which of the following is the most definitive therapy for this condition?

A) Topical application of corticosteroids
B) Systemic administration of antihistamines
C) Topical application of 5% permethrin cream
D) Systemic administration of corticosteroids
E) Typical application of wet dressings with Burow's solution

Endocrinology

60) Each of the following is more commonly associated with diabetes mellitus type 2 *EXCEPT* for:

A) Obesity
B) Hyperglycemia
C) Earlier age of onset
D) Treatment with metformin
E) The presence of acanthosis nigricans

61) Which of the following can be used to definitively distinguish diabetes melitis type 1 from type 2?

A) Family history of Type 2 diabetes
B) Serum C- Peptide level
C) Acanthosis nigricans
D) Diabetic ketoacidosis
E) Beta cell autoantibody level

62) You are evaluating a 16 year old boy who is obese, with dark velvety skin on his neck and chest and a family history of type 2 diabetes. His fasting glucose is 110 mg/dL and 2 hour glucose challenge test is 230 mg/dL. Which of the following is true regarding this patient?

A) He meets the American Diabetic association criteria for diabetes melitis
B) He should be started on a trial of metformin
C) He should be started on a trial of glyburide
D) Nutritional counseling and increased exercise followup if symptomatic
E) He does not meet the American Diabetic Association criteria for diabetes melitis and requires no further treatment of management.

63) In normal female pubertal development, which of the following represents the normal sequence?

A) Full Pubarche → Full thelarche → menarche
B) Partial Pubarche → Partial menarche → thelarche
C) Menarche → thelarche → Welder's arc
D) Full Thelarche → Full pubarche → menarche
E) Partial Thelarche → Partial pubarche → menarche

64) A mother wants to know when she can expect her 5 year old daughter to start her "periods." You tell her that, in addition to it being close to the time she herself started having her periods, environmental and nutritional factors have to be considered. The average American girl has her first period at what age?

A) 9-1/2
B) 10-1/2
C) 11-1/2
D) 12-1/2
E) 13-1/2
F) 16-1/2

65) There is a lot happening during the hormonal explosion of puberty which some blame on global warming. Everything seems to be flying out of the hypothalamic, pituitary highway. You of course know that all of the following levels are increased during puberty with the *EXCEPTION* of:

A) Water levels due to the polar ice cap melting
B) Insulin-like Growth Factor (IGF)
C) Thyroxine
D) Testosterone
E) Estrogen

66) During which Genital SMR stage does the growth spurt occur on average in boys?

A) SMR 1
B) SMR 2
C) SMR 3
D) SMR 4
E) SMR 5

67) During which Breast SMR stage does the growth spurt occur on average in girls?

A) SMR 1
B) SMR 2
C) SMR 3
D) SMR 4
E) SMR 5

68) Your patient is a 12 year old boy who, according to his family and teachers, has become increasingly more emotional and hyperactive and has not been able to sleep well at all. The symptoms have developed gradually over the past year and a half. You work in a small rural town that is not even recognized by your car's GPS. The nearest community hospital is roughly twice the size of your dashboard GPS.

On physical examination his TM's are clear, and mucous membranes moist. Eye grounds are normal with extraocular muscles intact (EOMI) with no exophthalmia. The rest of the exam is unremarkable. You suspect the patient is hyperthyroid. Which of the following is true regarding patients who are hyperthyroid:

A) Patients who are hyperthyroid can occasionally be jaundiced
B) The absence of exophthalmia rules out Graves's disease
C) Hepatomegaly is a common finding
D) Pretibial myxedema is a common finding in children who are hyperthyroid

69) Which of the following is the first sign of male pubertal development?

A) Axillary hair
B) Facial hair
C) Testicular enlargement
D) Peak growth velocity
E) Penile growth coupled with pubarche
F) Unwillingness to separate from his Cleveland Brown football helmet in mixed company

70) The first sign of pubertal development in females is:

A) Axillary hair
B) Pubarche
C) Hiding the Cleveland Brown helmet from their male counterparts
D) Thelarche
E) Menarche

71) In the following set of questions, decide if each numbered choice applies to (A) only, (B) only, both (C), or neither (D):

1) Delayed bone age
2) Normal adult height
3) Family history
4) Precocious puberty
5) Screened for newborns

(A) Hypothyroidism
(B) Constitutional growth delay
(C) Both
(D) Neither

72) For each number, choose the letter on the graph that best corresponds.

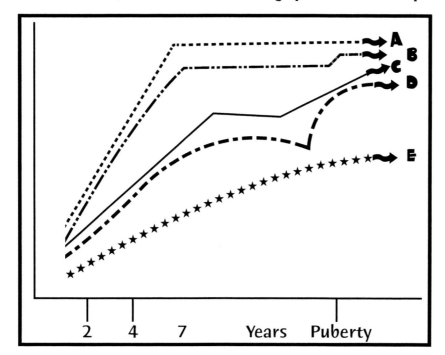

For the following questions, select the line on the graph that best corresponds to the correct diagnosis for short stature.

1) Craniopharyngioma
2) Hypothyroid
3) Untreated congenital adrenal hyperplasia
4) Constitutional delay
5) Genetic short stature

73)   For each number, choose the letter on the graph that best corresponds.

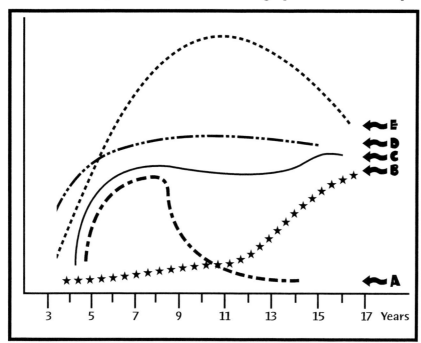

For the following questions, select the line on the graph that best corresponds to the correct mass or volume of tissue.

1) Blood volume
2) Spleen
3) Thymus
4) Testes
5) Skull

74a) You are presented with a 14-year-old girl whose height and sexual maturation differ from those of her peers. On physical examination, her height is lower than the 5%ile, and weight is in the 10%ile. Temperature is 37.1 C, HR is 72/minute, RR is 18, and BP is 95/67 in the arms and 105/86 in the legs. You note a broad chest, scattered pigmented nevi, and hyperconvex fingernails and toenails. Tympanic membranes are opaque and show decreased mobility. Tanner is stage 1 for breast development and stage 2 for pubic hair. Adnexa are difficult to assess on examination. A systolic ejection click is heard at the left lower sternal border.

At physical exam at birth, loose redundant skin around the neck and her records show a growth rate of decreasing velocity after 3 years of age. She also had frequent episodes of otitis media during childhood. Each of the following is likely to be associated findings EXCEPT:

A) 45, X Karyotype
B) Horseshoe kidney on renal ultrasound
C) 45, XXY Karyotype
D) Bicuspid aortic valve on cardiac echo
E) Pedal edema

74b) Each of the following would be appropriate medication for this particular patient EXCEPT:

A) Growth hormone
B) Oxandrolone
C) Medroxyprogesterone acetate
D) Estrogen
E) Listening to Tina Turner videos from the 80's

75) A 15-year-old underwent surgical resection of a suprasellar tumor. He was discharged from the hospital after one week. His hospital course was unremarkable. Ten days later he is experiencing lethargy coupled with dizziness. On physical examination his skin turgor is poor, eyes appear sunken, and he has orthostatic hypotension. Serum glucose concentration is 42 mg/dL. Serum sodium concentration is 124 mEq/L and serum potassium concentration is 6.1 mEq/L. Based on these findings, the MOST likely diagnosis is:

A) SIADH
B) Septic shock
C) Adrenal insufficiency
D) Cushing syndrome
E) Diabetes insipidus

76) Each of the following is a common complication of prednisone therapy EXCEPT:

A) Memory loss
B) Glucose intolerance
C) Growth retardation
D) Cosmetic effects
E) Increased risk for infection

77) The parents of a 10-year-old boy are concerned about their son's short stature. Height and weight are less than the 5%ile for age, and his growth velocity is 5 cm/year. The father is 64 inches tall, and the mother is 58 inches tall. Of the following, the MOST likely cause of this patient's short stature is:

A) Congenital adrenal hyperplasia
B) Hypothyroidism
C) Familial short stature
D) Growth hormone deficiency
E) Constitutional growth delay

78) You are asked by a boy's parents to estimate their son's adult height. Assuming that both parents' have reached their genetic potential, you tell them that the BEST estimate can be determined by:

A) Pulling a random number out of both parent's hats and dividing by 3
B) The mean parental height
C) The mean parental height plus 6.5 cm
D) The mean parental height minus 6.5 cm
E) Measuring the bone age at the onset of puberty

79) You are asked by a girl's parents to estimate their daughter's adult height. Assuming that both parents' have reached their genetic potential, you tell them that the BEST estimate can be determined by:

A) Pulling a random number out of both parent's hats and dividing by 3
B) The mean parental height
C) The mean parental height plus 6.5 cm
D) The mean parental height minus 6.5 cm
E) Measuring the bone age at the onset of puberty

80) A 16-year-old girl is concerned about her obesity. Menarche occurred at 12 years of age, and menstrual periods have been irregular. She has been otherwise healthy. Her height is at the 85%ile and weight >95%ile. She has moderate papulonodular acne and abundant facial hair. Which of the following is the MOST likely diagnosis?

A) Hypothyroidism
B) Exogenous obesity
C) Anabolic steroid abuse
D) Stein-Leventhal Syndrome
E) Gonadal dysgenesis

ENT

81) **An 8 month old presents to your office with suprasternal and subcostal retractions and inspiratory stridor. There is some improvement of the stridor with expiration. You explain to the parents that:**

A) Surgical correction will be needed
B) Direct laryngoscopy will be needed
C) A barium swallow is indicated to rule out extrinsic compression
D) No intervention is necessary at this time because this condition will improve with time
E) They should consider a career in "creative" yodeling for the child

82) **The diagnosis of otitis media is *BEST* made through:**

A) Mothers' insistence on antibiotics because they are leaving on a trip
B) Tympanometry
C) Pneumatic otoscopy
D) Viewing the tympanic membrane through the otoscope
E) D and C

83) **In the following set of questions, decide if each numbered choice applies to (A) only, (B) only, both (C), or neither (D):**

1) Inspiratory stridor   (A) Laryngomalacia
2) Expiratory stridor   (B) Tracheomalacia
3) Secondary to injury to the recurrent   (C) Both
   laryngeal nerve   (D) Neither
4) Status post tracheo-esophageal fistula repair

84) **All of the following are true statements regarding airway obstruction "above the glottis" EXCEPT:**

A) "Hot potato" voice can be a sign
B) Obstruction improves with expiration
C) It can present as a surgical emergency
D) It typically presents with expiratory stridor
E) High fever and drooling can be a feature

85) **A 3-year-old boy has a fever of 39.8C and severe respiratory distress. Three days prior to present illness, he developed rhinorrhea, a brassy cough, and a low-grade fever. He initially improved but has since been exhibiting more severe respiratory distress.**

On physical examination, he has stridor and retractions, along with decreased air entry. O₂ Sats are 90%. Lateral x-ray of the neck shows a normal epiglottis. AP views show a "shaggy" border of the tracheal air shadow. The MOST likely diagnosis is:

A) Bacterial tracheitis
B) Acute spasmodic croup
C) Viral croup
D) Foreign body aspiration
E) Croupier disease

The best treatment for this condition would include:

A) Dexamethasone
B) Racemic epinephrine
C) Cool mist
D) IV fluids
E) IV antibiotics

86) A 3-month-old presents with progressive noisy breathing "since birth". The parents note that the noise is loudest when the baby is feeding.

The baby is not hoarse, and there is no history of the baby turning blue or not breathing. Findings on physical examination reveal a mild inspiratory stridor at rest that improves when he is prone. X-ray of the neck and chest are obtained and read as normal. The MOST likely diagnosis is:

A) FB aspiration
B) Laryngomalacia
C) Tracheomalacia
D) Subglottic hemangioma
E) Laryngeal papillomatosis

87) Each of the following is true regarding *laryngotracheitis* EXCEPT:

A) It is also known as "viral croup"
B) Most cases occur in the early spring or late fall
C) Typical age of patient is 12 months
D) It has an abrupt onset with no preceding upper respiratory infection
E) Stridor is biphasic

88) You have in your practice a child with *acute otitis media with effusion*. The father is a microbiologist, and he wants to know the likely etiology. You would be correct in telling him that it could be any of the following EXCEPT:

A) *Haemophilus* influenza type B
B) Adenovirus
C) Streptococcus pneumoniae
D) Moraxella catarrhalis
E) Parainfluenza virus

89) **Each of the following is a true statement regarding laryngeal papillomas EXCEPT:**

A) Laser excision often needs to be repeated
B) Radiation treatment reduces the risk for malignant degeneration
C) It is acquired at birth from maternal vaginal condylomata
D) Surgery is not curative
E) They are not considered to be true neoplasm

90) **You are seeing a child for persistent middle ear effusion following two episodes of otitis media treated with antibiotics. Which of the following is true regarding the middle ear effusion?**

A) Inflammatory mediators play a role
B) Decreased blood flow to the mucous membranes is a factor
C) It is most likely due to persistent infection
D) Engorgement secondary to allergies is the likely cause
E) It is an indication for myringotomy tube placement

91) **A 7-1/2-year-old female presents with a periauricular mass of 9 months' duration. The mass is firm, non-tender. She is afebrile, and there is and has been no evidence of erythema or any other neck masses. The MOST likely diagnosis or etiology is:**

A) Psychogenic adenopathy
B) Atypical mycobacteria
C) Cat scratch fever
D) Neoplastic disease
E) Paramyxovirus

92) You are the attending in the ER, where you are presented with a 6-year-old boy with a 4-hour history of inspiratory stridor and a temperature of 38.1C. The parents have refused immunizations out of concern for the "increased risk for autoimmune disease". The child is apprehensive and leaning forward to facilitate breathing and you note that the child is also drooling. The MOST appropriate initial step would be to:

A) Obtain a lateral view x-ray study of the neck
B) Administer cefuroxime, 50 mg/kg IV
C) Request the presence of an individual skilled in intubation
D) Obtain an ABG
E) Examine the pharynx

93) Each of the following is true statements regarding acute otitis media except:

A) Daily antibiotic prophylaxis is a proven method to prevent recurrent otitis
B) The heptavalent pneumococcal vaccine has resulted in a drop in the incidence of OM due to S. pneumoniae
C) Exposure to passive smoke increases risk for recurrent OM
D) Children attending child care at increased risk for recurrent OM
E) The benefit of vaccine is higher in children older than 2 who have had at least one episode of OM

94) Which of the following would be an appropriate antibiotic to use for a dental infection in a 4 year old patient who is allergic to penicillin?

A) Azithromycin
B) Cipro
C) Penicillin
D) Clindamycin
E) A and D

95)   **Which of the following should alert the clinician to an intracranial complication of otitis media?**

A)   Hearing loss
B)   Otorrhea
C)   Otalgia
D)   Vomiting and blurred vision
E)   Rhinorrhea

96)   **Immediate treatment of focal swelling, pain and erythema of the pinna, following a traumatic event, consists of?**

A)   Ice packs
B)   Imaging studies
C)   ENT referral in 3-5 days after swelling has abated
D)   Head CT
E)   Evacuation of hematoma

97)   **Which of the following pathogens is the most likely cause of chronic sinusitis?**

A)   S. pneumoniae
B)   H. Flu type b
C)   Staph aureus
D)   Moraxella catarrhalis
E)   Group B strep

98)   **The SNAP[2] protocol has recently been used successfully to allow an ear infection to go 48 hours before parents will fill a prescription for antibiotics. Which of the following situations would prevent you from implementing this strategy?**

A)   Fever for 24 hours
B)   Symptoms of otitis media for 24 hours
C)   Another episode of otitis media in the past 3 months
D)   Children younger than 18 months
E)   No movement of tympanic membrane with insufflation

---

[2] Safety –net antibiotic prescription is what SNAP stands for.

99) A child with recurrent otitis media presents in your office. She also has had several episodes of pneumonia requiring hospitalization. Growth and development are normal. On physical exam there are no oral lesions, lungs are clear, heart sounds are normal, no thrills, murmur, or gallops, however the heart sounds are loudest on the right side.

Which of the following would be most helpful in establishing a diagnosis?

A) Cardiac echo
B) Measurement of serum immunoglobulin levels
C) Sweat test
D) Electron microscopic examination of nasal mucosa
E) HIV testing

ER

100) Each of the following may be administered via an endotracheal tube *EXCEPT* for:

A) Lidocaine
B) Epinephrine
C) Sodium bicarbonate
D) Atropine
E) Narcan

101) You are following an 8month old in the ER who initially presented with moderate respiratory distress. He has responded well to a series of albuterol treatments. Your decision to discharge him from the ER vs. admit him to the floor for additional treatment should take into account all of the following *EXCEPT* for:

A) Parental reliability
B) Paramyxovirus as the underlying cause
C) PO intake and hydration status
D) Use of racemic epinephrine while in the ER
E) Resolution of the symptoms after a period of observation

102) You are called to the ER where a mom and a 3 month old are waiting for you. Mom is in a custody battle in a nasty divorce[3] and she points to a red raised rash on the child's abdomen. Which may have been present at birth but "it is definitely worse, especially now after spending a week with his father". "Not only that," adds the grandmother as she walks in shaking off her umbrella on the code tray and your clogs, "look at the black and blue marks on his lower back and the one on his ankles." You notice that the black and blue marks are all the same color with no variation, and the raised red pattern is also not tender. You inform the mother, grandmother (grandfather who was staring at the wall the whole time) that:

A) You will document this clear case of paternal child abuse and cooperate with their attorney free of charge if necessary
B) The red rash is a strawberry hemangioma that will naturally get worse before it gets better, and the black and blue marks are Mongolian spots that they probably did not notice earlier. There is no abuse suspected
C) You will call Child Protective Services to document this and have them interview the mother to make sure it wasn't she who inflicted the damage and is only trying to cover herself
D) You join the grandfather and comment on the color of the wall.

103) Each of the following is often used in the treatment of acute methamphetamine intoxication **EXCEPT** for:

A) Phentolamine
B) Nifedipine
C) Beta blockers
D) IV normal saline
E) Lorazepam

104) A 5-year-old child is intubated and mechanically ventilated following respiratory arrest secondary to septic shock. Twenty-four hours later, his HR is 45 and BP is 135/105 mm Hg. The *most urgently* required intervention at this time would be:

A) 12-lead EKG
B) Vasodilators IV
C) Insertion of a central venous catheter
D) Lumbar puncture
E) Hyperventilation

---

[3] Is there any other kind?

105) A 16year-old girl is brought to the ED. She is comatose and unresponsive to verbal or painful stimuli. You start a normal saline bolus and secure her airway. Temperature is 35.8 C, with a heart rate of 65, respiratory rate of 6, and BP of 84/56. Muscle tone is flaccid. Pupils are equal but constricted. Blood glucose concentration is 225 mg/dL. The MOST appropriate next step would be to administer:

A) Naloxone
B) Physostigmine
C) Atropine
D) Atropine
E) Glucose

106) The *most serious* consequence of glue sniffing is:

A) Chronic rhinitis
B) Ataxia
C) Cardiac arrhythmia
D) Hallucinations
E) Lead encephalopathy

107) A 16-year-old boy is diagnosed with acute appendicitis, and emergency surgery is necessary. The patient is a chronic asthmatic on chronic oral steroids. He is also taking albuterol via nebulizer as needed and Pulmicort® daily via nebulizer.

The MOST appropriate management in anticipation of surgery would be:

A) Perform an ACTH stimulation test
B) Measure serum cortisol concentration
C) Measure serum glucose concentration
D) Begin high-dose inhaled corticosteroid therapy
E) Administer perioperative corticosteroids IV

108) Each of the following would be appropriate steps in managing hypokalemia EXCEPT:

A) Cardiorespiratory monitoring
B) Administration of potassium
C) Administration of insulin and glucose
D) IV fluids
E) Monitoring of acid – base balance

109) A 14-year-old has a two-day history of progressively worsening vomiting. In addition, the patient is complaining of chills and RUQ abdominal pain. WBC is 22,000. Urine Cx grows >100,000 colonies of *E. coli*/mL of urine. Which of the following is the MOST likely diagnosis?

A) Renal stones
B) Cystitis
C) Cholecystitis
D) Acute pyelonephritis
E) Gallstones

110) A 13-year-old boy who fell while skateboarding was unconscious for 5-7 minutes. He does not recall what happened immediately after he fell he is not complaining of a headache. He has vomited twice since the fall.

On physical exam, he is alert and oriented times three, with a Glasgow Coma Scale score of 14. There is no blood behind his tympanic membrane or nasal discharge. His neurological examination is within normal, as is the remainder of the physical exam. The MOST appropriate next step in managing this patient would be:

A) X-ray of the skull
B) Urinalysis
C) Abdominal ultrasound
D) CT scan of the head
E) Overnight observation; additional studies pending clinical status

111) A 17-year-old boy is brought to the ER by ambulance. He was found at home more disoriented and confused than usual.[4] He is ataxic with increased deep tendon reflexes. Muscle rigidity, increased salivation, and nystagmus are noted on physical exam. He is also exhibiting catatonic behavior. His BP is 170/100. Which of the following is the MOST likely diagnosis?

A) Phencyclidine intoxication
B) LSD intoxication
C) Opiate intoxication
D) Hyperventilation syndrome
E) Hysteria
E) Speaker of the house

112) A 13-year-old is brought to the ED directly from school after being "jumped" by several classmates. In addition to a sore arm and a hematoma noted on his forehead, he complains that his nose hurts and that he is having difficulty breathing. He is tender of the bridge of his nose, and there is marked swelling of the nasal septal noted, resulting in virtual occlusion of both nares. The *most appropriate* next step would be:

A) Head CT
B) X-ray of the nasal bones and zygomatic arch
C) Play the theme from new release of Rocky
D) Have him seen by ENT within one week once swelling has subsided
E) Evaluation by ENT as soon as possible

113) A 4-1/2-year-old lethargic child is brought to you from the triage area. The child has been doing well and the history is unremarkable. The child's mother is being treated for depression. Each of the following would be appropriate measures EXCEPT:

A) 12-lead EKG
B) Oxygen saturation monitor
C) Syrup of ipecac
D) Activated charcoal
E) Endotracheal intubation

---

[4] Even more than the disorientation and confusion that is baseline for the average teenager.

114) **Which of the following findings could have a likely explanation OTHER THAN child abuse?**

A) 6-month-old presenting with fussiness, tender leg, and metaphyseal fracture of the proximal tibia
B) 2-year-old with bruising on the shin and evidence of healed fractures on the same site secondary to falling on several occasions; child is very active
C) 3-year-old with rib fractures and who is taking ice skating lessons
D) 5-year-old with a skull fracture first noted in the morning by the parents
E) 3-month-old with soft tissue swelling of the face and jaw and evidence of cortical thickening of the long and flat bones

115) **Deferoxamine is administered IV to a child who ingested an unknown amount of ferrous sulfate. Shortly after administration, the urine has a pink color. The physiological explanation for this is that:**

A) Free serum iron has been chelated with deferoxamine and excreted in the urine
B) Insufficient iron was ingested to chelate all the deferoxamine, which is then excreted in the urine
C) Unbound serum transferrin has been chelated with deferoxamine and excreted in the urine
D) Hemoglobin-iron has been chelated with deferoxamine, causing hemolysis and hemoglobinuria
E) The serum iron concentration exceeds the chelating capacity of deferoxamine, allowing free iron excretion in the urine

116) **You are evaluating a 2 year old for the possibility of sexual molestation. The medical student working with you asks how who will ultimately decide whether sexual abuse has or has not occurred. The answer is:**

A) The examine pediatrician
B) A team of sexual abuse specialists
C) The court system
D) Child protective services
E) The police department

117) **The most common form of child abuse is:**

A) Emotional deprivation
B) Verbal abuse
C) Physical abuse
D) Sexual abuse
E) Neglect

118) **A mother reports by telephone her 4-year-old daughter fell from a wagon and hit her head on the sidewalk. The girl was unresponsive for one minute. She has vomited twice and is now sleepy but easily aroused. You would *most appropriately* advise the mother to:**

A) Keep the child quiet, administer aspirin for headache, and let her continue to sleep
B) Examine the child every hour for pupillary size and reactivity, and bring her to the ER if either pupil enlarges or reacts poorly
C) Bring the child to the hospital for careful clinical evaluation
D) Take the child to the hospital for x-ray study of the skull
E) Administer small doses of phenobarbital at home for the next 48 hours

119) **Which of the following is true regarding domestic violence in the home?**

A) Domestic violence occurs in 20% of households where children are abused
B) The incidence of domestic violence in the general population is 20%
C) There is a 150% increase in risk of child sexual abuse in households where domestic violence takes place
D) Comfort with a clinician could be a sign of domestic violence
E) In households that experience 50 or more episodes of domestic violence 10% of children will be physically abused by their mothers

120) Each of the following is true regarding the use of ketamine for conscious sedation *except:*

A) It produces sensory blockade
B) It can trigger "emergence hallucinations"
C) It decreases secretions
D) It is useful for short painful procedures
E) It is often used in conjunction with midazolam

121) Midazolam has each of the following characteristics *except* for:

A) Analgesic
B) Amnesic
C) Anxiolytic
D) Sedating
E) Enigmatic

122) Which of the following is the most likely trigger of life threatening anaphylaxis in children?

A) Snake bite
B) Bee sting
C) Food
D) MMR vaccine
E) Perfume

123) An afebrile 9 month old presenting with intermittent episodes of crampy abdominal pain with bilious vomiting. On physical exam you note right lower quadrant pain. In between episodes of pain the patient is reported to be lethargic. You note a "coiled spring" appearance on radiography.

The most likely diagnosis would be:

A) Your hallucinating the coiled spring out of a desire to pop a champagne bottle and retire
B) Swallowed foreign body
C) Cyclic vomiting syndrome
D) Intussusception
E) Abdominal migraine

Fluids & Lytes

124) You are evaluating an 8 week old boy. He is being breast-fed and you compliment the mother. However, she is also giving him chamomile herbal tea. She brought him in because he is "not himself" and seems a bit lethargic.

On physical exam, his TM's are non-injected, throat is clear, abdomen soft, lungs clear, and no murmurs are noted. He does appear to be severely dehydrated. You order the following labs: serum sodium 127 mEq/L, potassium 3.2 mEq/L, chloride mEq/L 73 mEq/L, bicarb 43 mEq/L, Bun/CRE 49/1.3. U/A is insignificant with a urine sodium of 5 mEq/L. The most likely etiology is:

A) Isotonic dehydration
B) Hyponatremic dehydration
C) Renal failure
D) Proximal renal tubular acidosis
E) Congenital adrenal hyperplasia

Which other test would be indicated in light of this?

A) Serum 17 hydroxylase
B) Serum 21 hydroxylase
C) 24-hour creatinine clearance
D) Sweat chloride
E) Skull X- ray

125) **Please match the diagnoses on the left with the lab values on the right**

			Na	K	Cl	Glucose	BUN	Urine Sp.Gr.Dx
1)	Lab error	(A)	152	4.3	118	95	28	1.002
2)	Pseudohyponatremia	(B)	152	4.2	119	73	22	1.020
3)	Hyponatremic dehydration	(C)	122	4.0	90	76	4	1.029
4)	SIADH	(D)	121	4.2	84	80	20	1.021
5)	Hypernatremic dehydration	(E)	122	4.2	107	450	10	1.017
6)	Diabetes insipidus	(F)	119	4.3	105	80	10	1.011

126) **A 20-month-old infant who has congenital heart disease is currently receiving digoxin and furosemide. Which of the following sets of drug-related conditions are most likely to develop in this patient?**

A) Hyponatremia and hyperkalemia
B) Hypernatremia and hyperkalemia
C) Hyperchloremia and hypokalemia
D) Hypernatremia and hypokalemia
E) Hypochloremia and hypokalemia

127) **Which of the following is best represented by an arterial pH of 7.35, PCO2 of 30 mm Hg, PO2 of 110 mm Hg, and a serum bicarbonate concentration of 18 mEq/L?**

A) Respiratory acidosis with metabolic compensation
B) Respiratory alkalosis with metabolic compensation
C) Metabolic alkalosis with respiratory compensation
D) Respiratory acidosis with respiratory compensation
E) Metabolic acidosis with respiratory compensation
F) Lab error

128) **A 6-month-old infant has a 5-day history of producing 13 to 14 stools a day, mostly watery diarrhea. He has a blood pressure of 55/35 mm Hg, heart rate of 170, RR of 55, and is afebrile. The peripheral pulses are palpable but weak and his skin is cold and mottled. The patient is producing urine. After successfully starting an IV, your NEXT step would be to:**

A) Congratulate yourself for starting an IV on such a "difficult stick"
B) Administer D_5 0.45% Normal Saline 10 cc/kg over 20 minutes
C) Administer ringers lactate 20 cc/kg over 20 minutes
D) Administer D_5 0.2% Normal Saline 20cc/kg over 10 minutes
E) Hold off on fluid administration pending intubation
F) Administer oral rehydration

129) **A 2% concentration of glucose (111 mmol/L) in solution for oral rehydration is chosen because at this concentration:**

A) Coupling of intestinal sodium transport is optimal
B) Secretory diarrhea is prevented
C) Hypoglycemia is prevented
D) Hepatic glycogen stores are adequately replaced
E) Insulin secretion is appropriately reduced

130) **A 9-year-old has a serum sodium concentration of 125 mEq/L 4 hours after an admission to the PICU for a head injury. Fluid intake via IV has been appropriate, yet urine output has been only 0.7 to 1.0 mL/kg/hr. On physical examination he appears euvolemic, and neurological findings have remained unchanged since admission. The central venous pressure will be maintained at 5-7 cm H_2O. In addition, you should consider:**

A) Infuse a 3% saline solution at 1% of body weight over 1 hour
B) Change fluids to an isotonic saline solution at maintenance rate of infusion
C) Reduce of fluid administration to 2/3 maintenance
D) Infuse a 5% albumin solution at 1% of body weight
E) Infuse 0.5 g/kg of mannitol

131) Which of the following are ignored during calculation of plasma osmolality?

A) Sodium
B) Chloride
C) Potassium
D) Bicarb
E) BUN

132) Each of the following is observed in patients with congestive heart failure *except* for:

A) Increased body weight
B) Hypernatremia
C) Edema
D) Abnormal salt retention
E) Normal serum osmolality

133) A 9 month old child presents with poor weight gain over the past 5 months. Weight and height are below the 10th percentile for age. The child is afebrile with stable vital signs and the infant appears to be thin on physical examination.

Lab findings include:

Sodium	134
Potassium	4.0
Chloride	115
Bicarb	16
VBG	7.25
PCO2	28
Urine pH	7.1

Which of the following is most consistent with this patient's clinical presentation?

A) Pulmonary hypertension
B) Inborn error of metabolism
C) Renal tubular acidosis
D) Diabetic ketoacidosis
E) Alcoholic ketoacidosis

134) Each of the following is a cause of metabolic alkalosis *except* for:

A) Laxative abuse
B) Organophosphate poisoning
C) Diuretic therapy
D) Gitelman syndrome
E) Bartter syndrome

135) Each of the following is an adverse consequences of severe alkalemia *except:*

A) Arteriole constriction
B) Reduction in coronary blood flow
C) Hypoventilation
D) Hypocapnia
E) Hypokalemia

136) You are evaluating a 7 week old male with increasing severity of projectile vomiting until now where he cannot tolerate any PO feeds without forceful vomiting.

Lab studies include:

Sodium – 130
Potassium – 3.5
Chloride – 90
Bicarb 35

Which of the following is likely to reveal the underlying disorder?

A) Plain x-ray
B) 17 hydroxy (OH) progesterone level
C) Abdominal ultrasound
D) pH probe study
E) Air contrast enema

137) **Which of the following is characteristic of heat stress?**

A) Decreased exercise performance
B) Confusion
C) Nausea and vomiting
D) Core temperature between 100.4 F and 104 F
E) Core temperature greater than 104 F

Genetics

138) **Each of the following are associated with a delayed eruption of teeth *EXCEPT* for:**

A) Gardner's syndrome
B) Hypothyroidism
C) Hypopituitarism
D) Ectodermal hypoplasia
E) NHL hockey syndrome

139) **Each of the following symptoms are associated with Treacher Collins syndrome *EXCEPT* for:**

A) Small jaw
B) Mental retardation
C) Ear abnormalities
D) Lower eyelid abnormalities
E) Conductive hearing loss

140) **All of the following are inherited in an autosomal dominant inheritance pattern *EXCEPT* for:**

A) Waardenburg syndrome
B) Aicardi syndrome
C) Retinoblastoma
D) Tuberous sclerosis
E) Achondroplasia

141) **Edwards Syndrome (Trisomy 18) is associated with all of the following *EXCEPT* for:**

A) Hypoplastic nails
B) Rocker bottom feet
C) Bicornate uterus
D) Prominent occiput
E) Horseshoe kidney

142) **A couple in your practice is expecting their first child. Mom has myotonic muscular dystrophy and they would like to know the odds of this child having the disorder. You tell them:**

A) 50% if the child is male and 0% if the child is female.
B) 25%
C) 50%
D) 100%
E) It is the same as the general population

143) **Patau syndrome (Trisomy 13) is associated with each of the following EXCEPT:**

A) Scalp defects
B) Congenital heart defects
C) Rocker bottom feet
D) Microphthalmia
E) Holoprosencephaly

144) The chances of an asymptomatic girl, whose brother has Cystic Fibrosis, being a carrier is closest to:

A) 0%

B) 33%

C) 25%

D) 66%

E) 100%

145) You are in the Delivery room and have attended a routine C/Sxn, and suspect the baby has Down's syndrome. Mom is 24 years old and did not have an amniocentesis and therefore does not suspect any problem. All the following will increase your index of suspicion for Down's syndrome *EXCEPT* for:

A) Cleft lip/palate

B) Wide gap between first and second toe

C) Duodenal atresia

D) Redundant skin, posterior neck

E) Palmar simian crease

146) It is December 26th and you have 40 patients in your waiting room not counting the ones you are actually evaluating in your examination rooms. You get an e-mail from the Department of Public Health. One of the patients in your practice has been identified as "positive PKU" (phenylketonuria). In addition to diet counseling and placing this infant on Lofenalac®, you need to order the following:

A) A Thriller Vanilla Lofenalac® cocktail for yourself tonight (Lofenalac® and vanilla Absolute® vodka)

B) Serum NH_4 every 6 months

C) Anion gap and B12 levels

D) Homocysteine levels

E) Testing for tetrahydrobiopterin deficiency

147) The parents of one of your patients would like to know the odds of their having a child with hemophilia A. The father has a brother with the disorder but he himself is unaffected.

A) 0%
B) 25%
C) 50%
D) 100%
E) 125%

148) The pattern of inheritance of myoclonic epilepsy is *BEST* described as:

A) Occurring through patrilineal inheritance
B) Occurring through matrilineal inheritance
C) X-linked inheritance patterns
D) Due to abnormalities in mitochondrial DNA
E) D and B

149) A 9 year old boy is well known to your practice because he is very friendly whenever he comes to the office and speaks a lot, although content is lacking. His physical exam is most notable for small hands, feet, and genitalia. He was noted to be floppy as an infant. Genetic studies would reveal:

A) Trisomy 13
B) Deletion on chromosome 13
C) Deletion on chromosome 15 inherited from his father
D) Deletion on chromosome 15 inherited from his mother
E) You identify this as Bill Clinton, pass GO and collect $200

150) Which of the following *BEST* describes the inheritance pattern of tuberous sclerosis?

A) X-linked recessive
B) X-linked dominant
C) Autosomal dominant
D) Autosomal recessive
E) Random mutation

151) In the following set of questions, decide if each numbered choice applies to (A) only, (B) only, both (C), or neither (D):

1) Pulmonic stenosis
2) Coarctation of the aorta
3) Webbed neck
4) Chromosomal abnormality
5) Can affect females

(A) Turner's syndrome
(B) Noonan syndrome
(C) Both
(D) Neither

152) You are at a cocktail party enjoying the appetizers and decent California white wine with an excellent bouquet. The word is out that you are a doctor and some investment banker with a lot less personality than the wine's bouquet pulls you aside and says, "Doc, I have a question. My sister is going to marry a guy whose brother has cystic fibrosis. She doesn't have it. What are the chances of their having a kid with cystic fibrosis?" Your answer is:

A) 1 in 4
B) 1 in 20
C) 1 in 150
D) 1 in 200
E) How the heck do I know? I am not a geneticist, now how about some stock tips you creepy loser?

GI

153) **A 2-1/2 year old child with a history of failure to thrive and frequent loose stools. Giardia has been ruled out. Your presumptive diagnosis is gluten-sensitive enteropathy. The definitive test to diagnose gluten-sensitive enteropathy is:**

A) Have the child attend the annual Gluten and Garlic festival and watch the results from the reviewing stand
B) The gluten challenge test
C) A serum antigliadin antibody measurement
D) A small bowel biopsy

154) **Which of the following is consistent with a diagnosis of chronic non-specific diarrhea in the toddler?**

A) Flatulence that has guests leaving on schedule.
B) Normal growth
C) Bloody stools
D) Severe abdominal pain
E) Vomiting

155) **You are asked to be one of the keynote speakers at the "Passing the boards without passing a stool" conference. The title of your lecture is "Chronic Diarrhea, Will It Get you in the End?" After describing the stool velocity and splatter patterns, you describe the hallmarks of the stool found in chronic non-specific diarrhea in the toddler. Your list, consistent with a diagnosis of chronic non-specific diarrhea in the toddler, is correct with the _EXCEPTION_ of:**

A) Stool pH less than 5 and positive reducing substances
B) Occult blood
C) Rarely passing stools during sleep
D) Mostly occurring in the morning
E) Watery diarrhea

156) **Match the GI condition on the left with the clinical description on the right.**

1) Fecal impaction
2) Partial small bowel obstruction
3) Crohn's disease
4) Mesenteric venous obstruction

(A) Bloody diarrhea followed by seizure
(B) Malodorous green stools with fever
(C) Left lower quadrant fullness
(D) Pressure tenderness on the right lower quadrant along with fever and joint aches
(E) Teen using oral contraceptives
(F) Vomiting, weight loss and anorexia

157) **In the following set of questions, decide if each numbered choice applies to (A) only, (B) only, both (C), or neither (D):**

1) Skipped lesions are common
2) Associated with ankylosing spondylitis
3) Surgery is curative

(A) Crohn's disease
(B) Ulcerative colitis
(C) Both
(D) Neither

158) **A 5-month-old infant presents with poor weight gain and a voracious appetite. The parents note that the child has foul smelling greasy stools that "require a gas mask", according to the parents.[5] On physical examination you note a rather small, thin infant that also appears to be pale. You politely confirm the parents' assessment of the stool as you discretely dispose of it through a trap door you create *with your bare hands* on the spot.**

You obtain a CBC, which reveals a low white blood cell count and a low hematocrit. You obtain two negative sweat chloride tests. Incidental x-ray finding reveals metaphyseal dysostosis. Which of the following is the MOST likely diagnosis?

A) Cystic fibrosis
B) Diamond-Blackfan syndrome
C) Inflammatory bowel disease
D) Metaphyseal dysplasia
E) Shwachman-Diamond syndrome

---

[5] Foul-smelling stools are often described, yet isn't this redundant? Are there any other kinds of stools?

159) Which of the following approach is MOST appropriate with uncomplicated gastroesophageal (GE) reflux?

A) Barium swallow
B) PH probe sleep study
C) 24-hour apnea monitoring at home
D) Pulmonary consultation
E) Observation over time

160) The MOST common symptom of gastroesophageal (GE) reflux in infants is:

A) Projectile vomiting
B) Recurrent regurgitation
C) Apnea
D) Epigastric abdominal pain
E) Poor weight gain
F) Aspiration pneumonia

161) Which of the following is BEST associated with tocopherol deficiency?

A) Megaloblastic anemia
B) Photophobia and blurred vision
C) Glossitis
D) Hemolytic anemia
E) Poor wound healing

162) Anorexia, slowed growth, drying and cracking of the skin, hepatosplenomegaly, and increased intracranial pressure would MOST likely be the result of an EXCESS of:

A) Niacin
B) Ascorbic acid
C) Riboflavin
D) Cyanocobalamin
E) Retinol

163) Deficiency of cyanocobalamin can be associated with each of the following conditions EXCEPT:

A) Homocystinuria
B) Juvenile pernicious anemia
C) Celiac disease
D) Methylmalonic aciduria
E) Dermatitis

164) Match the numbered causes of infantile vomiting with the lettered descriptions on the right.

1) GER (gastroesophageal reflux)   (A) Does not occur during sleep
2) Rumination   (B) Polyhydramnios
3) Necrotizing enterocolitis   (C) Normal phenomenon in nearly all infants
4) Duodenal atresia   (D) 10% to 35% of the affected infants are full term

165) Match the numbered *cause of vomiting* with the lettered *description on the right.*

1) Neurological etiology   (A) Rapid drop in hematocrit
2) Gastroesophageal reflux   (B) Associated with weight loss, hypoalbuminemia, and diarrhea
3) Rumination   (C) May present with chronic respiratory problems and rhinitis
4) Gastrointestinal cow milk allergy   (D) Can occur with posturing
5) Allergic gastroenteropathy   (E) May respond to behavioral interventions

166) Each of the following is true regarding Wilson disease *except* for:

A) Autosomal dominant
B) Can present with a mixed conjugated and unconjugated hyperbilirubinemia
C) It is rarely manifests before age 3
D) Trientine , a copper chelator is one form of treatment
E) Zinc acetate which prevents absorption of copper from the GI tract is another form of treatment

167) **Each of the following are possible complications of GERD in infants except**

A) Feeding refusal
B) Poor weight gain
C) Apnea
D) Anemia
E) Upper airway symptoms

168) **Each of the following statements regarding Rotavirus is true *except:***

A) The primary mode of transmission is fomite
B) It is mostly seen during the winter
C) Rotavirus has been isolated from the respiratory tract
D) Delayed gastric emptying plays no role in vomiting seen during acute infection
E) Adults are more likely to be asymptomatic

169) **Each of the following is true regarding abdominal migraines *except:***

A) It is more common in males
B) It can present as episodic epigastric pain
C) It can present as episodic periumbilical pain
D) Family history is often present
E) Acute episodes can last an hour or more

GU

170) A 4-year-old girl is having difficulty with toilet training. The parents report that their daughter has constant dribbling of urine during the day and night. On examination, urine appears to be draining from the vagina. Results of urine analysis and culture are normal. Which of the following is the MOST likely diagnosis?

A) Diabetes insipidus
B) Neurogenic bladder
C) Giggling incontinence
D) UTI
E) Ectopic uretal orifice

171) A 17-year-old boy had a unilateral orchidopexy for a cryptorchid testis when he was 10 years old. He now seeks further information. You would tell him most appropriately that:

A) Retractile testicles without intervention can result in cryptorchidism
B) Surgical correction clearly decreases the overall risk of malignancy
C) Self-examination of the testes on a regular basis is particularly important post-op
D) Boys with a retractile testis are at increased risk for infertility or malignancy
E) There is no cause for concern because operative correction was successful

172) You are evaluating a 2 month old boy for his routine physical exam. The baby's development has been progressing nicely; he is in the 50th percentile for height, weight and head circumference. The father who is in the 95th percentile for bad taste in T shirts and jeans is very concerned about the size of his son's penis. You measure the boy's penis and note it to be 4.1 centimeters and both testes are descended.

The most appropriate next step in managing this patient would be:

A) Ask the father why the obsession with his son's penis size
B) Obtain a CT scan of the head
C) Obtain a genetic karyotype
D) Measure serum 17-hydroxy progesterone
E) Delicately reassure the father

173) During a routine physical examination of an 18 month old you are unable to palpate the left testicle despite the documentation of bilateral descended testicle during previous visits.

The most appropriate next step in evaluating this patient would be:

A) Testicular ultrasound
B) Trial of HCG shots
C) Urological consult
D) Reposition and re-examine the patient
E) Transilluminate the scrotum

174) A 16-year-old girl presents in the ER at 1:00 AM, reporting that she has had intermittent mild abdominal pain and nausea for 10 days. She states that menses have been regular since menarche over 3 years ago. Her physical exam is unremarkable. UA reveals Sp. gravity of 1.010, a trace of glucose, no protein, and 2-3 WBC/HPF. The MOST appropriate next step would be to order:

A) VCUG
B) Barium enema
C) IVP
D) Urine human chorionic gonadotropin
E) Glucose tolerance test

175) Which of the following is true regarding acute testicular pain?

A) The blue dot sign distinguishes testicular torsion from torsion of the testicular appendage
B) Torsion of the testicular appendage requires cold compresses and immediate surgical excision
C) Nausea and vomiting are the hallmarks of epididymitis
D) True bacterial epididymitis is rare in children
E) Inguinal hernia never results in acute scrotal pain

Heme One

176) Each of the following are associated with tumor lysis syndrome *EXCEPT* for:

A) Hyperphosphatemia
B) Hyperkalemia
C) Hypernatremia
D) Hyperuricemia
E) Alkalinization treatment

177) Each of the following are characteristic of Hodgkin's lymphoma *EXCEPT* for:

A) Reed-Sternberg cells
B) Rapidly growing non-tender abdominal mass
C) Non tender cervical nodes
D) Elevated white blood cell count
E) Low lymphocyte count

178) By definition, neutropenia in a 6 year old child is an absolute neutrophil count of less than:

A) 400
B) 1500
C) 2500
D) 3500
E) 4500

179) A father with G6PD deficiency has a daughter who presented to the ER with dark urine. The girl is pale and lethargic. The *BEST* explanation for this is:

A) Munchausen Syndrome by Proxy (MSBP)
B) A new mutation
C) Father is a carrier
D) Mother is a carrier
E) Father has the disorder and mom is a carrier

180) A 3 year old presents with a history of recurrent stomatitis, lymph node enlargement, and one episode of clostridium perfringens pneumonia. You suspect a diagnosis of cyclic neutropenia. What interval between neutropenic phases would help you confirm the diagnosis?

A) 1 week
B) 3 weeks
C) 24 weeks
D) 36 weeks
E) 6 months – 1 year
F) A millennium plus or minus a century

181) Please match the association on the left with the diagnosis on the right.

1) Lysosomal granules   (A) Chediak-Hitachi syndrome
2) Chronic Staph infections   (B) Chronic granulomatous disease
3) Delayed separation of the umbilical stump (C) Cyclic neutropenia
4) Clostridium perfringens   (D) Leukocyte adhesion deficiency
5) Pancreatic insufficiency   (E) Shwachman-Diamond syndrome

182) In the following set of questions, decide if each numbered choice applies to (A) only, (B) only, both (C), or neither (D):

1) Low iron binding capacity
2) Low serum ferritin
3) High serum ferritin
4) Low MCV, low RDW

(A) Anemia of chronic illness
(B) Iron deficiency anemia
(C) Both
(D) Neither

183) In the following set of questions, decide if each numbered choice applies to (A) only, (B) only, both (C), or neither (D):

1) X-linked recessive
2) Autosomal dominant
3) Mucosal bleeds

(A) Hemophilia A
(B) Hemophilia B (Christmas disease)
(C) Both
(D) Neither

184) In the following set of questions, decide if each numbered choice applies to (A) only, (B) only, both (C), or neither (D):

1) Uncommon in African Americans
2) History of trauma
3) Pain worse at night, relieved by ibuprofen
4) Eats a lot of donuts, works in the safety department at a nuclear reactor and is cerebrally challenged

(A) Ewing's sarcoma
(B) Osteogenic sarcoma
(C) Both
(D) Neither

185) In the following set of questions, decide if each numbered choice applies to (A) only, (B) only, both (C), or neither (D):

1) Normocytic anemia
2) Macrocytic anemia
3) Affects the red cell line primarily
4) Primarily occurs in the newborn period
5) Spontaneous recovery
6) Primarily seen in toddlers

(A) Transient erythroblastopenia of childhood
(B) Diamond Blackfan syndrome
(C) Both
(D) Neither

186) A 1-year-old boy has been less active for the past 3-4 days with decreased PO intake. With the exception of a URI 3 weeks earlier, he has done well. His physical exam the boy is afebrile with vital signs stable except for notable pallor the rest of the physical exam is unremarkable.

His labs include a WBC of 7.3, ANC of 100, H/H of 18/6, and MCV of 80. His platelet count is 352 K with a retic count of 0.1%. The MOST likely diagnosis is:

A) G6PD deficiency
B) Sickle cell anemia
C) Diamond-Blackfan anemia
D) Acquired aplastic anemia
E) Transient **erythroblastopenia**
F) Iron deficiency

187) A 2-year-old boy is brought to you for an evaluation because he has been walking with an unsteady gait and occasionally exhibits "seizure-like activities" such as random eye movements and "myoclonic" movements. An abdominal mass is noted on physical examination.

The MOST likely preliminary diagnosis is:

A) Cerebral palsy
B) Trauma secondary to child abuse
C) Wilms' tumor
D) Neuroblastoma
E) Myoclonic seizure disorder

188) With regard to anemia of chronic illness, all of the following are true Except:

A) Serum ferritin level is elevated
B) Serum iron binding capacity is reduced
C) Marrow iron stores are decreased
D) Mean corpuscle volume (MCV) is reduced
E) Anemia is improved with treatment of the underlying condition

189) **A 16-year-old girl is due to have a dental extraction. Her history is significant for menorrhagia and prolonged oozing following a similar dental procedure a year ago. Before going ahead with this procedure, one would be best advised to:**

A) Administer platelets and fresh frozen plasma prior to the procedure
B) Have the dentist increase his coverage limits on her malpractice policy
C) Administer Factor VIII and titrate to achieve appropriate hemostasis
D) Before proceeding, do a coagulation workup to rule out von Willebrand's disease
E) Before proceeding, do a coagulation workup to rule out Factor VIII deficiency

190) **A 3-year-old boy has been seen for chronic seborrheic dermatitis of the scalp of worsening severity. In addition, there is concern over polydipsia, polyuria, and discharge from his ear.[6] Realizing that this is not simply seborrheic dermatitis, you diagnose:**

A) Seborrheic dermatitis with secondary infection
B) Severe combined immunodeficiency
C) Wiskott-Aldrich syndrome
D) Stevens-Johnson syndrome
E) Langerhans' cell histiocytosis

191) **Which of the following dermatological disorders would be of MOST concern regarding malignant transformation?**

A) Ichthyosis vulgaris
B) Strawberry hemangioma
C) Incontinentia pigmenti
D) Xeroderma pigmentosum
E) Acanthosis nigricans

192) **Which of the following neoplasms shows the strongest familial tendency?**

A) Osteosarcoma
B) Congenital hepatoma
C) Retinoblastoma
D) Wilms' tumor
E) Acute lymphoblastic leukemia

---

[6] Poly otorrhea, if you will.

193) An 8-year-old boy with sickle cell disease has had abdominal pain, nausea, and vomiting for 8 hours. He has had similar pain intermittently over the past 5 months. Usually the pains subsided after 3-4 hours. When you examine him, you note that he is afebrile, slightly jaundiced, and that there is upper quadrant abdominal tenderness. Which of the following is the MOST appropriate next step in evaluating this patient?

A) Upper gastrointestinal endoscopy
B) X-ray of the abdomen
C) Barium swallow
D) Ultrasound of the gallbladder
E) Exploratory laparotomy

194) The *most common* indication for a transfusion in a patient with hereditary spherocytosis would be:

A) Extramedullary hematopoiesis
B) Aplastic crisis
C) Severe fatigue
D) Hypersplenism
D) Growth retardation

195) Which of the following statements is true regarding the inheritance pattern of hereditary spherocytosis?

A) It is primarily X linked recesssive
B) It is primarily X linked dominant
C) It is primarily autosomal recessive
D) It is primarily autosomal dominant
E) It is rarely seen in people of Northern European descent

196) **Which of the following is true regarding splenectomy in children with hereditary spherocytosis?**

A) Partial splenectomy is of no benefit
B) Splenectomy should be done prior to age 5 to be of any benefit
C) Splenectomy is indicated for patient's wanting to participate in contact sports
D) The risk of infection is highest one year after splenectomy
E) Prophylactic penicillin is of no benefit.

197) **Treatment with which of the following chemotherapeutic agents increases the risk for developing bladder cancer as a *secondary malignancy?***

A) Anthracycline
B) Etoposide
C) Ifosfamide
D) Cyclophosphamide
E) Methotrexate

198) **Before treating a child for folate deficiency one must first exclude B12 deficiency and document folate deficiency by:**

A) Serum folate levels
B) Mean corpuscle volume
C) Segmented neutrophils
D) Erythrocyte folic acid concentration
E) Reticulocyte count

199) You are evaluating a patient with hyperpigmented patches and are below the 10th percentile for both weight and height. On physical exam you also note that the patient has thumbs which can best be described as non-functional and small.

The most likely explanation for the findings would be:

A) Bloom syndrome
B) Rubinstein Taybi syndrome
C) Thrombocytopenia absent radius
D) Fanconi anemia
E) Osteogenic sarcoma

200) You are evaluating a 16 year old girl whose last menstrual period was 3 weeks ago. She denies sexual activity and her urine pregnancy test is negative. She has intermittent right lower quadrant pain for 6-8 weeks. You order a pelvic ultrasound which reveals multiple ovarian cysts measuring less than 2 cm.

The most appropriate next step in managing this patient would be:

A) Obtain a Serum BHCG
B) Renal ultrasound
C) Amylase and lipase
D) Abdominal CT with oral and IV contrast
E) Serum tumor markers to rule out ovarian cancer

ID

201) You are treating a child for Lyme disease documented on serological study, with oral amoxicillin. The child now presents with a high fever with severe chills. Mom reports to your office as a drop-in appointment to find out "why you are not treating this correctly". You tell her:

A) She is correct. You are treating "Lime" disease not "Lyme" disease; without a medical spell checker you are lost!
B) You will switch the child's medication to doxycycline, the optimal choice.
C) You will administer a shot of IM ceftriaxone and increase the dosage of amoxicillin
D) This is consistent with treatment

202) An 11 year old child reports to your office on Monday morning. He has just returned from a trip with his grandfather to New Mexico. The boy is proudly wearing the Daniel Boone hat his grandfather gave him. For three days the boy has had fever, muscle aches and the "worst headache" he has ever had in his life. On physical exam you note a macular rash that does note blanche with pressure. The rash is on his wrists, ankles, palms and soles. On closer exam you notice that some of the rash appears to be petechial and purpuric. Your next step is to:

A) Obtain a blood culture, CBC, and appropriate serological studies, and schedule a followup visit next week if things do not improve
B) Obtain a CBC, blood culture, and IM ceftriaxone, and schedule a close followup visit
C) Note that the Daniel Boone hat is actually a live skunk that is asleep and politely (and very quietly) usher him to the isolation room
D) Start a full course of chloramphenicol
E) Start a full course of doxycycline

203) A diagnosis of mumps is consistent with each of the following *EXCEPT* for:

A) Negative mumps specific IgM
B) Aseptic meningitis
C) Bilateral orchitis
D) Pancreatitis
E) Unilateral orchitis

204) Because of your dynamic personality, dapper clothing, and eccentric tastes in red wine, you are called to speak to the local PTA on tuberculosis. They want to know the best way to tell if their child has TB. You tell them:

A) Night sweats
B) Positive skin test
C) High fever
D) Fatigue
E) Painful cough

205) Which of the following drugs used in the treatment of tuberculosis is associated with optic neuritis?

A) Ethambutol
B) Pyrazinamide
C) Rifampin
D) Isoniazid
E) Streptomycin

206) A 5-year-old girl presents with two red papules on her right arm. On physical examination the child has a temperature of 38.5C, has a poor appetite, and is complaining of a headache. Prominent lymph nodes are noted in the right axilla. There is also a maculopapular rash on his trunk and conjunctivitis of the left eye. History is significant only for his playing in the back yard at a friend's house 2 weeks ago. The *most likely* diagnosis is:

A) Rocky Mountain spotted fever
B) Kawasaki disease
C) Rubeola
D) Bartonella henselae infection
E) Pasteurella multocida infection

207) In the following set of questions, decide if each numbered choice applies to (A) only, (B) only, both (C), or neither (D):

1) Pharyngitis with exudate
2) High fever, enlarged tonsils
3) Hepatosplenomegaly
4) Atypical neutrophils
5) Group A beta hemolytic strep +

(A) Infectious mono
(B) Strep pharyngitis
(C) Both
(D) Neither

208) A 3-year-old girl presents with fever, cough, abdominal pain, and poor appetite for one week. She has also been complaining of diarrhea. On physical exam you note an enlarged spleen and "rose spots" on the abdomen and thighs. Which of the following tests should be ordered *first* in further evaluation of this patient?

A) *Salmonella* agglutinins
B) Blood culture
C) Widal test
D) Peripheral blood smear
E) Abdominal CT

209) A 9-month-old infant has had a fever with a T max of 39.2C along with bloody diarrhea that lasted for 2-3 days. You are seeing the infant for followup later that week. The infant is now afebrile. Stool cultures taken at the time of illness are now positive for *Salmonella* species. A blood culture taken at the same time is negative. Treatment with which of the following would be MOST appropriate?

A) Amoxicillin
B) Trimethoprim /sulfamethoxazole therapy
C) Ceftriaxone
D) Amoxicillin clavulanic acid
E) Observation

210) A 12-year-old has been exposed to a classmate at school who was positively diagnosed with *Streptococcal* pharyngitis. Which of the following is the MOST appropriate recommendation to the parents?

A) The girl should be removed from school for one week
B) The girl should be treated with penicillin and return to school 24 hours after starting treatment
C) Throat cultures should be obtained from all children in the girl's class, treatment pending culture results
D) A throat culture should be obtained from the girl if any symptoms of a *Streptococcal* infection appear
E) The girl should receive IM Bicillin®

211) Corticosteroids would routinely be indicated in the management of which of the following conditions?

A) Infectious mononucleosis
B) Kawasaki disease
C) Tuberculosis meningitis
D) Acute urticaria
E) Toxic shock syndrome

212) **Each of the following is true regarding infantile botulism EXCEPT:**

A) Constipation is a late finding
B) Gentamicin should never be used.
C) Botulism toxin blocks the release acetylcholine from the presynaptic neuron
D) Botulism toxin is the active ingredient of Botox® injections
E) Treatment is largely supportive.

213) **A child with which of the following would appropriately be excused from attending their first-grade class tomorrow?**

A) Diffuse rash secondary to roseola
B) Infectious mono
C) Tinea corporis 48 hours after the start of Griseofulvin
D) *Strep* throat and fever
E) *Asymptomatic Salmonella gastroenteritis*

214) **After visiting his uncle last month, a 7 year-old boy presents with fever, muscle aches, and a headache. In addition, you note severe conjunctivitis and preauricular lymphadenopathy. Serological testing confirms infection with *Francisella tularensis*. Which of the following antibiotics could be used to treat this boy? :**

A) Vancomycin
B) Tetracycline
C) Doxycycline
D) Ciprofloxacin
E) Gentamicin

215) **In order to reduce the risk for ototoxicity of gentamicin, you would:**

A) Obtain a level 30 minutes after the first dose
B) Obtain a level 30 minutes after the third dose
C) Obtain a level 30 minutes prior to the second dose
D) Obtain a level 30 minutes prior to the fourth dose
E) Gauge it on appropriate dosing and clinical response

216) It is 4 AM and you are covering the pediatric ER, and you just "cleared the charts"[7] from the rack. Your next patient is well known to you since it is a 4-year-old who has chronic paronychia infections. The most likely cause of this chronic infection is:

A) The desire of this family to make sure you do not sleep while on call
B) *Pseudomonas aeruginosa*
C) *Staph aureus*
D) *Candida albicans*
E) Group A beta-hemolytic *Strep*

217) You are now board certified, and in order to maintain hospital privileges you have been assigned to the infection control committee and must now lecture the residents, medical students, and senior members of the housekeeping staff. You correctly tell them that each of the following requires *droplet precautions* EXCEPT for:

A) Pertussis
B) Mumps
C) Croup
D) Pneumococcus
E) Rubella

218) A boy in your practice is being treated for meningococcemia. In addition to appropriate antibiotic treatment, which of the following additional measures would be the MOST appropriate?

A) Immunization of contacts with meningococcal vaccine
B) Oral administration of rifampin to family members
C) Oral administration of sulfadiazine to family members
D) Assessment of splenic function in the patient during convalescence
E) Assessment of adrenal function in the patient during convalescence

[7] As in no more patients in the waiting room.

219) A 3- year -old child presents with rhinorrhea, fever, conjunctivitis, and pharyngitis. What is the MOST likely diagnosis?

A) Adenovirus
B) Beta-hemolytic *Strep*
C) Epstein-Barr virus
D) *Staph aureus*
E) *Haemophilus influenzae* type b

220) An 18-month-old has a one-week history of cough, tachypnea, diminished PO intake and appetite, and now presents with a 2-day history of high fever. On physical exam, the child is grunting and retracting with some abdominal distension. CXR shows a right middle lobe infiltrate with a large pleural effusion. Which of the following organisms is the MOST likely cause of this patient's disease?

A) Mycoplasma pneumoniae
B) *Chlamydia pneumoniae* (TWAR)
C) Adenovirus
D) Staph aureus
E) *Moraxella Catarrhalis*

221) A 15-month-old child presents with a generalized rash for 3 days with a temperature of 38.1 °C. On physical exam, you note generalized tender erythematous skin with denuding of the skin over parts of the trunk, with the base of each of these areas appearing to be clear and shiny. You also notice flaccid bullae with crusting around the mouth and nose. Physical findings are otherwise normal. Which of the following is the most likely diagnosis?

A) Erythema multiforme major
B) Staphylococcal scalded skin syndrome
C) Epidermolysis bullosa
D) Bullous impetigo
E) Kawasaki syndrome

222) You are called upon to take care of a 4-year-old boy who is HIV positive. He presents with weight loss, malaise, abdominal pain, and diarrhea. Prior to this he has been asymptomatic. Management of HIV infection is unknown. By isolating which of the following pathogens would you be MOST justified in diagnosing AIDS?

A) *Salmonella* species
B) *Mycobacterium avium* complex
C) *Campylobacter* species
D) Streptococcus pneumoniae
E) Haemophilus influenzae

223) A 12-year-old boy presents with a 1-day history of pain in his right thigh. On physical exam, his temperature is 39.3C with a HR of 110 and RR of 34. Pain is noted with palpation of the distal portion of his affected thigh and on movement of the right knee. However, there is no swelling or effusion noted on his knee. His CBC is remarkable for a WBC of 17,500 mm^3 with a left shift. ESR is 51. Which organism is the MOST likely guilty party?

A) *H flu* type b
B) Group B beta-hemolytic *Strep*
C) Staphylococcus aureus
D) *Salmonella* species
E) Gnu painus

224) Following treatment for H. pylori gastritis which of the following would be valid tests to document the eradication of the pathogen?

A) Fecal H. pylori antigen
B) Endoscopy with biopsy
C) Urease breath test
D) H. pylori IgG
E) A,B,C

225) You are caring for a child who attends day care with a child who is in the pediatric intensive care unit for meningococcal sepsis. The child and the family left on vacation 5 days ago, which was the last day the child was in the same classroom with the index case.

The story has made national news and the parents saw it on CNN and are calling you for advice. Your advice to them is:

A) Seek medical attention if the child develops fever or a rash
B) The child and parents need chemoprophylaxis
C) The child needs chemoprophylaxis
D) Stop watching CNN and start watching the Daily Report with Jon Stewart.
E) Since the child was exposed 5 days ago no intervention is needed

226) Which of the following is true regarding treatment of children with Hepatitis C?

A) All patients respond equally to Ribavirin monotherapy
B) All patients respond equally to Interferon and Ribavirin
C) Response to treatment is dependent on the viral genotype
D) Patients with genotype 1 do not respond to treatment
E) Patients with genotypes other than type 1 do not respond to treatment

227) You are evaluating a 7 year old child who presents with a papular rash on the trunk along with several vesicular lesions on his trunk. The papular rash has now developed on the face and extremities. One day prior to development of the rash he developed a fever of 102.3. His immunization status is unknown.

He cannot return to school without a definitive documented diagnosis. Which of the following tests would help establish the correct diagnosis in the shortest period of time?

A) Viral culture
B) Molecular amplification
C) Skin biopsy
D) Direct fluorescent antibody
E) Polymerase chain reaction

228) You are treating a 12 year old with a community acquired skin infection which has not responded to treatment with cephalexin. You suspect the infection is due to a methicillin resistant Staph aureus infection. Which one of the following antibiotics would be most appropriate for this patient?

A) Amoxicillin/clavulanic acid
B) Cefdinir
C) Doxycycline
D) Levofloxacin
E) Amoxicillin

229) Which one of the following is the most appropriate *rapid* test for influenza virus?

A) Direct fluorescent antibody
B) Enzyme immunoassay antigen detection
C) Viral culture
D) Serum IgM titers
E) Polymerase chain reaction

230) Which of the following antibiotics would be *least* effective in treating Listeria monocytogenes?

A) Chloramphenicol
B) Penicillin
C) Trimethoprim-sulfamethoxazole
D) Cefotaxime
E) Gentamicin

231) Which of the following is true regarding CMV disease in patients receiving a stem cell transplant?

A) Latent CMV infection reactivates only if the donor is seropositive
B) Latent CMV infection reactivates only if the recipient is seropositive
C) Latent CMV infection reactivates if the donor *or* the recipient are seropositive
D) Latent CMV infection reactivates only if the donor *and* the recipient are seropositive
E) Reactivation quickly reverts to latent disease and is subclinical

232) Each of the following would be appropriate steps for a CMV seronegative pregnant mother to take regarding the care of her other child who is younger than 3, except *for:*

A) Sleeping in the bed should be completely eliminated
B) No kissing on or near the child's mouth
C) No changing of diapers or handling the child's laundry
D) Assume that any child younger than 3 years of age is secreting CMV in their saliva and urine
E) No sharing towels or washcloths with the child

233) Which one of the following would be most appropriate routine confirmation of cat scratch disease in a child?

A) Lyme node biopsy and culture
B) Wound culture
C) Antigen skin testing
D) Enzyme immunoassay (EIA)
E) Polymerase chain reaction

234) Which of the following is true regarding rabies in humans?

A) Prior rabies immunization provides protection against CNS disease
B) The diagnostic test of choice is direct fluorescent antibody staining
C) The diagnostic test of choice is reverse transcriptase-polymerase chain reaction
D) More than 50% of cases may have no documented history of exposure
E) The presence of high CSF rabies titers confirms previous disease

235) Which of the following would be the most appropriate treatment of a child bittern by a bat that was not isolated?

A) Reverse transcriptase-polymerase chain reaction testing
B) Wash the wound and treat with cephalexin only
C) Infiltrate the wound with rabies immunoglobulin
D) Provide HDCV today and on days 3,7,14, and 28
E) C and D

236) You are presented with a patient whose HBsAb is positive. The HBsAg, HBcAb total and IgM are negative. What is the correct interpretation of these results?

A) I am sorry I have to read the question again
B) Chronic hepatitis B infection
C) Chronic hepatitis C infection
D) Immune after recovery from hepatitis B infection
E) Immune following hepatitis B vaccine

237) Which of the following is associated with a low hepatitis B viral replication rate?

A) HBeAb
B) HBeAg
C) HBsAb with positive HBcAb
D) HBsAb with negative HBcAb
E) HelpmeIhavenoideawhattheansweris

Metabolic

238) The parents of a child with Wolman's disease need to be concerned with all of the following *EXCEPT* for:

A) Excessive total body triglyceride and cholesterol levels due to a defect in their breakdown
B) Calcified adrenal gland
C) Failure to thrive
D) Increased lifetime risk for cardiac disease due to increased serum triglyceride and cholesterol levels
E) Hepatosplenomegaly

239) In the following set of questions, for each numbered word or phrase, choose the lettered heading that is MOST CLOSELY ASSOCIATED with it. Lettered headings may be selected once, more than once, or not at all.

1) "Mousy odor" urine
2) "Sweaty sox odor" urine
3) Hypertonic and tachypneic during first week of life
4) "Dark urine"

(A) Isovaleric acidemia
(B) Alcaptonuria
(C) Maple syrup urine disease (MSUD)
(D) PKU

240) In the following set of questions, decide if each numbered choice applies to (A) only, (B) only, both (C), or neither (D):

1) Elevated serum ceruloplasmin
2) Elevated serum copper levels
3) Acute hepatic failure
4) Treated with IM penicillin
5) Elevated tissue copper levels
6) X-linked

(A) Wilson's disease
(B) Menkes Kinky Hair Syndrome
(C) Both
(D) Neither

241) A 3 1/2-week-old infant presents with fever, vomiting, a bulging fontanelle, and hepatomegaly. Jaundice and vomiting first presented during the second week of life. She has been breast-fed exclusively. Which of the following is the *most likely* diagnosis?

    A) Fructose aldolase deficiency
    B) Fructose-1, 6 biphosphate deficiency
    C) Glycogen storage disease type 1
    D) Neonatal adrenoleukodystrophy
    E) Galactosemia

242) A child born with which of the following disorders is at GREATEST risk for experiencing a cerebral vascular accident?

    A) Maple syrup urine disease
    B) Pompe disease
    C) Pompous disease
    D) Homocystinuria
    E) Hunter syndrome

243) You are evaluating a 5-month-old infant for poor weight gain and intermittent vomiting of several weeks' duration. Three weeks ago the infant was weaned from breast milk and started on cow milk, baby food vegetables, and fruits.

On physical examination you note that the infant is irritable, and jaundiced, with a liver palpable 3-4 cm below the right costal margin. Which of the following is the *most likely* diagnosis?

    A) Hypothyroidism
    B) Galactosemia
    C) Hereditary fructose intolerance
    D) Sensitivity to beta lactoglobulin
    E) Glycogen storage disease type 1

244) You are evaluating a boy with swelling of his left knee although he has not sustained any trauma. He has not been outdoors much, is afebrile and also is complaining of red eyes with no discharge. The rest of the physical exam is benign.

Which of the following other complaints or physical finding would you expect to see in this patient can you expect to elicit on taking a detailed history?

A) Kayser Fleisher rings
B) Malar rash
C) Dysuria
D) Evidence of physical abuse
E) Evidence of self mutilation

245) Elevated creatinine phosphokinase concentrations would be consistent with which of the following diagnoses?

A) Systemic lupus erythematosus
B) Duchenne's muscular dystrophy
C) Psoriasis Arthritis
D) Dermatomyositis
E) Wolman's disease

246) Soy formula would be most appropriate in a child with which of the following conditions?

A) Maple syrup urine disease
B) Pompe disease
C) Allergic colitis
D) Cow milk allergy
E) Galactosemia

247) You are evaluating an 18 month old boy whose growth and development are blunted. He is hypotonic with hepatosplenomegaly. You note a retinal cherry red spot on funduscopic exam.

The most likely diagnosis is:

A) Tay Sachs disease
B) Niemann Pick disease
C) Wolman disease
D) Wilson disease
E) Autism

Musculoskeletal

248) A frantic mother and her neighbor bring a 2 1/2 year old to your office in an ambulance. She has had hip pain for the past 2-3 days but does not appear to be ill. You comfort the child by giving him a stuffed Spongebob Squarepants doll.

While examining her you are able to move her hip through some flexion and abduction. She has a fever of 38.1°C, and the mother notes that he recently had a cold and cough. Lab results include a WBC of 11.2 with an ESR of 22. The ultrasound report indicates fluid in the affected hip. You suggest:

A) Aspiration, culture of the hip and broad-spectrum antibiotics pending definitive identification of an organism
B) Drainage of the hip, hospital observation, and bone scan
C) Rest, reassurance, ibuprofen and outpatient follow-up
D) MRI and oral antibiotics

249) A 3 year old boy brought to your office. His father, who at first glance appears to actually have no neck., requests braces because his kid is "walking like a pigeon" and will interfere with his football career. He notes that he had the same problem and had bars every night and this "set him straight". You suggest:

A) The father seek counseling and Prolixin Decanoate intramuscular IM for one month under psychiatric supervision
B) Ballet classes for father and son, and laughingly suggest no "bars" are needed, including the ones the father apparently visits on a nightly basis.
C) Denis-Browne bars every night to correct this problem that should have resolved by 18 months
D) Reassurance that the problem with resolve with time without the aid of bars and devices

250) A one-day-old neonate has tenderness and crepitus over the right clavicle. The remainder of the exam is normal. An x-ray study confirms a fracture of the mid portion of the right clavicle. Which of the following is the most accurate statement regarding this patient's condition?

A) Open reduction is required for treatment
B) Erb palsy will likely be present as well
C) Initial treatment and definitive treatment consists of securing the sleeve to the front of the shirt
D) A shoulder spiker is the treatment of choice
E) Pneumothorax is seen with this injury

251) A newborn male is noted to have disproportionately short limbs as well as a small chest. He has multiple healed fractures as well as new fractures of the long bones and ribs. Which of the following disorders would account for these findings?

A) Achondrogenesis
B) Fibrochondrogenesis
C) Thanatophoric dysplasia
D) Juvenile osteochondroses
E) Osteogenesis imperfecta
F) Trifecta imperfecta

252) A 2-year-old presents to the ED because of refusal to use his left arm. The child is afebrile with no evidence of trauma on physical examination. The left elbow is noted to be flexed, with the forearm in a pronated position. There is no swelling or discoloration, although the child is reluctant to allow you to examine the arm. The MOST appropriate next step is to:

A) Order and x-ray of the elbow
B) Order a bone scan
C) CBC, blood culture, and start antibiotics
D) Apply a splint and refer to ortho
E) Supinate the forearm while the elbow is flexed

253) Surgical intervention would be indicated in scoliosis with a curvature of:
A) 10 degrees
B) 20 degrees
C) 30 degrees
D) 40 degrees
E) depending on clinical manifestations

254) A 13-year-old boy is sent to you by his coach because of pain and swelling below his left knee. He is active in sports, particularly running, baseball, and skiing. Physical examination reveals joint tenderness over the anterior tubercle of the left knee. Which of the following is the most likely diagnosis?

A) Patellar dislocation
B) Osteochondritis dissecans
C) Tear of the collateral ligament
D) Osgood-Schlatter disease
E) Tear of medial meniscus
F) Overzealous throwing of a discus

255) A 12-year-old girl has a 7-week history of pain in the right heel. For the past 4 weeks she has also had pain in the left heel, the left calf, and the Achilles tendon. The pain worsens with walking.

The patient has been excused from all physical activity at school, including opening and closing her locker. She now refuses to walk, claiming that her leg is "paralyzed." She is afebrile and presents with no other symptoms.

On physical examination, the patient appears to be well but is somewhat uncomfortable and frequently shifts her position while seated but cannot move the left leg. Muscle tone and reflexes of the left leg are normal; the leg can be moved passively without pain or discomfort. Physical exam is otherwise unremarkable. Of the following, the most appropriate next step in the evaluation of this patient's condition would be:

A) Begin administration of nonsteroidal inflammatory drugs
B) Measure antinuclear antibody titers
C) Order x-ray studies of both lower extremities
D) Elicit additional history
E) Obtain an electromyogram

256) Osteomyelitis can spread locally to cause septic arthritis. After which age does is this risk reduced?

A) 6 months
B) 12 months
C) 36months
D) 48 months
E) closure of the growth plate

257) Which of the following differentiates clubfoot from metatarsus adductus?

A) Putting your foot in your mouth (figuratively of course)
B) Inability to dorsiflex the ankle with metatarsus adductus
C) Inability to dorsiflex the ankle with club foot
D) Positive Babinski with club foot
E) Negative Babinski with club foot

258) The definition of scoliosis is:

A) A spinal curvature on a posterior-anterior x-ray ,greater than 10 degrees
B) A spinal curvature on an anterior-posterior x-ray greater than 10 degrees
C) A spinal curvature on an posterior –anterior x-ray greater than 25 degrees
D) A spinal curvature on an anterior-posterior x-ray greater than 25 degrees
E) Based on clinical findings and pulmonary function

259) Duchenne muscular dystrophy is due to the absence of dystrophin which results in:

A) Muscle membrane instability
B) Nerve transmission disfunction
C) Neuromuscular junction blockade
D) Increased acetylcholine presynaptic uptake
E) Replacement of dystrophin with collagen

260) You are caring for a family where there is a child with Duchenne muscular dystrophy DMD. There is no prior family history and the molecular genetic testing in the child is negative. The risk for recurrence is closest to:

A) 0%
B) 10%
C) 25%
D) 90%
E) 100%

261) Congenital talipes equinovarus (club foot) is typically diagnosed by:

A) Cribside clinical diagnosis
B) CT scan
C) MRI
D) Ultrasound
E) Bone Scan

262) If conservative measures to treat congenital talipes equinovarus (club foot) are unsuccessful when should surgical interventions be implemented?

A) When the child begins to walk
B) When the child enters school
C) During pubertal development
D) During the first year of life
E) When the growth plates fuse

Neonatology

263) A full term, small-for-gestational-age baby is born to a 25 year old G3 P1 Mom. There was no prolonged rupture of membranes (PROM) and the mom is group B strep negative. She has received good prenatal care. The baby was born 4 hours ago and is being breast-fed, yet remains somewhat irritable jittery and tachypneic. Since it is 3 in the morning you are also irritable and jittery so you stop by the vending machine to pick up a couple of Kit Kats® to tide you over. You arrive and give a physical exam, which is unremarkable, but the neuro exam is positive for bilateral 5-10 beat ankle clonus. The first thing you should do at this point is:

A) Order a head ultrasound because, given the neurological findings, CNS asphyxia is very likely
B) Order a full sepsis workup and start ampicillin and gentamicin without delay
C) quit your job immediately (the hours and the Kit Kats ® are horrible) and sign a non-compete 30-year agreement with this infant as your agent, because clearly he has rhythm and is the next "Counting Crows" Ben Ulrich
D) Check the serum glucose and get ready for a D10 W bolus
E) Get some more Kit Kats® and microwave granola bars; it's gonna be a long night and morning

264) The most appropriate antibiotic regimen for empiric treatment of neonatal sepsis in the NICU setting is:

A) Ampicillin
B) Gentamicin
C) Cefotaxime
D) Ampicillin and gentamicin
E) Ampicillin and cefotaxime

265) An infant in your practice with Cystic Fibrosis is being supplemented with medium chain triglycerides (MCT). When, on rounds, you are asked why, you correctly answer:

A) Chain rhymes with sane and gets things through
B) MCT is partially water-soluble and can be directly transported into the portal vein.
C) Micelle formation is facilitated by MCT
D) Absorption in the distal small bowel is facilitated
E) Because of its stimulatory effect on bile acid production and secretion

266) A newborn is cyanotic with each feeding, which resolves as soon as the feeding stops. You strongly suspect choanal atresia and order the definitive test to make the diagnosis:

A) Skull films
B) Head CT
C) Attempt to pass an NG and confirm position with chest film
D) A feeding of pureed sea conch imported from the Cayman Islands; looked good on the "Learning Channel"
E) Head ultrasound

267a) A 2-week old infant has become increasingly irritable and been feeding poorly. He has a maculopapular rash on his trunk as well as hepatosplenomegaly. An ophthalmological exam reveals some inflammation of the retina. Head CT reveals some calcifications. The *MOST LIKELY* diagnosis is:

A) Toxoplasmosis
B) Congenital CMV
C) Congenital syphilis
D) Herpes simplex
E) Child Abuse

267b) This is *BEST* diagnosed with:

A) Head CT
B) Serum IgM
C) Serial serology measurement
D) Urine culture
E) Brain biopsy and EEG

268) Match each number (infant reflex) to the age on the right when it disappears under normal conditions:

1) Palmar grasp   (A) 2 months
2) Plantar grasp   (B) 4 months
3) Automatic stepping   (C) 6 months
4) Moro reflex   (D) 9 months
5) Money grasp   (E) Law school grad

269) In the following set of questions, decide if each numbered choice applies to (A) only, (B) only, both (C), or neither (D):

1) Resolves within 6 weeks
2) Positive Tensilon® test

(A) Transient myasthenia gravis (newborn)
(B) Congenital myasthenia gravis
(C) Both
(D) Neither

270) A full-term child is born to a 28-year-old mother with moderately controlled diabetes. Each of the following are complications of infants of diabetic mothers EXCEPT:

A) Maternal pyelonephritis
B) Congenital anomalies
C) Persistent pulmonary hypertension
D) Polycythemia
E) Hypercalcemia

271) A 32-hour-old baby with an Apgar of 9/9, who had been feeding well and appeared healthy up until now, has developed intermittent episodes of cyanosis. The oxygen saturations are in the high 50s with no improvement with oxygen supplementation. The infant does not appear to be in respiratory distress. The most appropriate NEXT step would be:

A) Start IV antibiotics
B) Endotracheal intubation
C) Cardiac echo
D) Start IV prostaglandins
E) Start IV indomethacin

272) An otherwise healthy newborn presents with persistent bilious vomiting at 24 hours of age. The MOST appropriate next step in managing this patient would be:

A) Abdominal ultrasound
B) Rectal stimulation to induce a bowel movement
C) Rectal exam and stool guaiac
D) NG tube, NPO, and 24-hour observation
E) Abdominal x-ray

273) An 18-month-old toddler who is being evaluated for the first time since birth has developmental delay, strabismus, chorioretinitis, probable hearing loss, and microcephaly. The mother is an unmarried teen who lives with her grandparents[8]. During the 4th month of pregnancy the mother had an illness characterized by lymphadenopathy. She cares for a pet cat in her home. Essential testing at this time would include each of the following EXCEPT:

A) Screening for congenital syphilis
B) X-ray of the skull
C) Developmental assessment
D) Evaluation for visual acuity
E) TORCH titers

274) Diffuse intracranial calcifications are documented. The patient also has documented hearing loss and active chorioretinitis. Each of the following would be appropriate steps in the management of this patient EXCEPT:

A) Administration of folic acid
B) CBC, and differential and platelet count
C) Administration of folinic acid
D) Pyrimethamine
E) Corticosteroids

---

[8] Yes that would be the child's great-grandparents

275) **Of the following, the neonate at greatest risk of developing infection with hepatitis B is a neonate whose mother:**

A) Received immune globulin
B) Was treated for preeclampsia
C) Recently had a blood transfusion
D) Is a recent immigrant from Lichtenstein
E) Is a drug user

276) **A healthy infant is born by forceps delivery in the breech position. At 9 days of age, she is brought for evaluation because of skin lesions. Mother's prenatal history is negative. Which of the following findings is *most likely* to require immediate hospitalization?**

A) Flat bluish discoloration over the posterior spine and buttocks
B) Scattered vesicles with erythematous bases confined to the buttocks
C) Pustular melanosis
D) Hard nodules with erythematous overlying skin confined to the lateral buttocks
E) Pigmented macules

277) **You are evaluating a 3-hour-old infant who is the product of an uncomplicated full term gestation vaginal delivery. With the exception of some grunting and a prolonged terminal labor, the delivery was an uncomplicated spontaneous vaginal delivery. The respiratory rate is 43 with no respiratory distress at this time. The hands and feet are noted to be cyanotic; otherwise the physical examination is within normal limits. The *most* appropriate next step in managing this infant would be:**

A) Obtain a CXR
B) Measure the arterial blood gas
C) Request a cardiology consultation
D) Administer oxygen via nasal canula
E) Place the infant under a radiant warmer

278) Which of the following BEST explains what is measured by a prenatal non-stress test?

A) Evaluates how much stress the average neonatal fellow can endure during the month of July
B) Evaluates the response of the infant's HR to drug induced uterine contractions
C) Evaluates fetal lung maturity
D) Evaluates the fetal autonomic nervous system integrity
E) Evaluates the volume of amniotic fluid present

279) You are evaluating a 3 day old infant who presents with abdominal distension without emesis. A KUB reveals large dilated loops of bowel with no air noted in the rectosigmoid area. On physical examination the anus is patent.

The most appropriate study in this scenario is:

A) Upper GI series
B) Endoscopy
C) Contrast enema
D) Abdominal ultrasound
E) Abdominal CT

280) A one month old male infant is brought in by a frantic father because of enlargement of both breasts[9]. He even has noted some milky white substance from the breasts and he tells you "when they said the milk would come down in 3 weeks is this what they meant?"

The prenatal and birth history are normal. Throughout the pregnancy mom took prenatal vitamins and acetaminophen for back pain and headache. On physical examination the baby is alert and interactive, appears to be well nourished with vital signs stable. Prominent breast buds are noted with no inflammation or erythema. You note bilateral descended testicles and normal genitalia. Which of the following is the most appropriate next step?

A) IV antibiotics
B) Skull x-ray
C) Reassurance
D) Review father's medication and diet
E) Review of maternal medications and diet

---

[9] In the baby not the father

281) **You are evaluating a 5-week-old infant who has lost weight since birth. On physical examination, he seems thin and you obtain the following lab values:**

Sodium of 135, potassium of 3.2, chloride of 102, and serum bicarb of 8. Arterial blood gas reveals a pH of 7.22 and a PCO_2 of 28. The *most likely* diagnosis would be:

A) Pulmonary disease
B) Distal renal tubular acidosis
C) Proximal renal tubular acidosis
D) Polycystic kidney disease
E) Maple syrup urine disease

282) **A full-term infant is born via normal spontaneous vaginal delivery. Very thick particulate meconium is noted. The baby is crying vigorously and has a one-minute Apgar of 8. The delivery was precipitous, leaving no time for the gynecologist to do DeLee suctioning on the perineum. You are attending the delivery as the pediatrician.[10] Which of the following would be the MOST appropriate management in this situation?**

A) Since the one-minute Apgar is 8, endotracheal intubation is not necessary
B) Since the one-minute Apgar is not 8, direct visualization via neither laryngoscopy nor endotracheal intubation is necessary
C) Direct visualization via laryngoscopy is indicated
D) Endotracheal intubation and suctioning to remove meconium are indicated
E) Due to the clinical status, no intervention is indicated

283) **You are performing a routine exam of a 6-month-old baby who was born at 32 weeks gestation. You would expect to find the following:**

A) Sit unsupported, babble, recognize strangers
B) Able to sit when supported only, rolls from back to stomach, smiles and laughs spontaneously, moves head appropriately toward sounds
C) Crawls, uses pincer grasp, waves
D) Keeps hand fisted, follows objects past midline, recognizes the parent
E) Pulls to stand, babbles, transfers objects when prompted

---

[10] As opposed to the videographer.

284) A very frantic nurse and mother call you to the nursery. A one-day-old infant has a rash that is concentrated on the trunk. The rash started out as papules but is now yellow, with pustules surrounded by red skin. The infant is doing well, except for anxiety. Maternal history is unremarkable. Upon further evaluation you would likely find:

A) A high WBC on CBC left shift and bacteremia
B) A high WBC on CBC predominately eosinophils
C) Wright stain of the lesion with primarily neutrophils
D) Wright stain of the lesion with primarily eosinophils
E) Tzanck smear with intranuclear inclusions

285) During prenatal screening, an elevated alpha-fetoprotein level is noted. Each of the following are legitimate concerns EXCEPT:

A) Twins
B) Omphalocele
C) Open spina bifida
D) Trisomy 21
E) Congenital nephrotic syndrome

286) Each of the following are associated with dietary protein intolerance in children *except:*

A) IgE mediated food hypersensitivity
B) Typically involves, egg, soy and mild proteins
C) Vomiting and diarrhea
D) Heme positive stools
E) Failure to thrive

287) Hypochloremic, hypokalemic metabolic alkalosis would be seen in:

A) Congenital adrenal hyperplasia
B) Pyloric stenosis
C) Protein intolerance
D) Gastroesophageal reflux
E) Intussusception

Neurology

288) While you are on rounds a child is presented with acute lateralized weakness and, since you haven't slept since the first season of American Idol ®, your "differential" is limited to "acute stroke". The ward-attending physician is appalled and asks you to do 5 pushups over a bedpan suspended by a fish line held by the medical students. With each pushup you are to shout each diagnosis in the differential. You will have redeemed yourself if you call out each of the following *EXCEPT*:

A) Todd postictal paralysis
B) Hemiparetic seizures
C) Subdural hemorrhage
D) Hypocalcemia
E) Hypoglycemia

289) A 10 month old presents with rapid onset hypotonia, lethargy and constipation. Mom states that no new foods have been introduced into the infant's diet. On physical exam, in addition to lethargy and hypotonia, you note mydriasis and diminished reflexes. This disorder would *BEST* be diagnosed with:

A) Head CT
B) Head MRI
C) Karyotype
D) Tensilon test
E) EMG

Primary treatment would be:

A) Gentamicin
B) Tensilon
C) Ampicillin and ceftriaxone
D) Immunization update
E) Supportive

290) You are in the ER, at 4:30 in the morning and have to counsel the anxious parents of a child who has experienced a simple febrile seizure. The parents want to know the *BEST* way to prevent any future such occurrences. You tell them:

A) Diazepam at the onset of fever
B) Continuous anticonvulsant therapy
C) Intermittent anticonvulsant therapy
D) Anticonvulsant therapy if the febrile seizure recurs
E) Antipyretics as soon as the fever presents

291) A 6 year old girl diagnosed with mild mental retardation presents with a history of intermittent seizures. She also has a history of infantile spasms. On physical exam, you note microcephaly and several hypopigmented patches distributed over her body along with a fleshy bump near her nose. This disorder would *BEST* be diagnosed with which study?

A) Head CT
B) Head MRI
C) Karyotype
D) EEG
E) EMG

292) In the following set of questions, decide if each numbered choice applies to (A) only, (B) only, both (C), or neither (D):

1) Can involve the eyes
2) Progressive onset
3) Treatment is curative
4) Prevented with immunization

(A) Infantile botulism
(B) Myasthenia gravis
(C) Both
(D) Neither

293) Match the diagnosis on the left with the clinical history on the right.

1) Structural headaches   (A) Pain in the neck or shoulders
2) Migraine   (B) Aggravated by sneezing, coughing, or straining
3) Tension headache   (C) Cyclic vomiting and recurrent abdominal pain

294) A 10-year-old boy was diagnosed with migraine headaches one year ago. His headaches have been treated with ibuprofen. Over the past few weeks he has been complaining of early morning headaches, often severe enough to wake him up. There has been a lot of academic pressure at school according to the parents. He has also vomited before breakfast in the morning.

On physical examination, you note that his fundi are normal, and that he has mild lower extremity hyperreflexia. The gait is normal and tone and strength are equal and symmetric. Which of the following is the MOST appropriate next step?

A) Order MRI of the head
B) Order an EEG
C) Refer to a psychologist for anxiety management
D) Suggest eating breakfast first thing in the morning
E) Consider beta blockers to control performance anxiety rather than ibuprofen

295) You examine a full-term infant with a head circumference of 39 cm. You would be correct in informing the family that the child has:

A) Macrocephaly
B) Microcephaly
C) Craniosynostosis
D) Normocephalic
E) Beckwith-Wiedemann syndrome

296) You are presented with an infant who is exhibiting multifocal clonic seizure. Multiple attempts to control it with multiple doses of phenobarbital have failed. You review the EEG tracing and stroke your beardless chin.[11] You appear to be concentrating deeply even though, to your untrained eye, the EEG looks no different than the geological society tracing of a typical earthquake. However, Lenny, your neurology consultant informs you that it is a "paroxysmal pattern of generalized bursts of bilaterally synchronous high-voltage activity intermixed with spikes or short waves". The MOST likely explanation for these clinical findings and the EEG tracing would be:

A) Herpetic encephalitis
B) Confirmation of your suspicion that Lenny is a fraud, since this actually was a geological tracing of an earthquake you showed him
C) Pyridoxine dependency
D) Hypoxic-ischemic encephalopathy
E) Intracranial hemorrhage

297) A 3-month-old boy has had constipation and weakness for 5 days. He is alert but has drooping eyelids, sluggishly reactive pupils, and decreased reflexes. Findings on physical exam are otherwise normal. Which of the following is the *most likely* diagnosis?

A) Myasthenia gravis
B) Muscular dystrophy
C) Spinal muscular atrophy (Werdnig-Hoffmann disease)
D) Poliomyelitis
E) Infantile botulism

---

[11] We are referring to female physicians here of course.

298) You are evaluating a 10 year old girl who has been experiencing headaches for the past few weeks. The headaches are primarily occipital accompanies by a spinning sensation, ringing sound, double vision and difficulty maintaining balance.

The headaches occur several times per week and in between headaches she is asymptomatic. The neurological exam is unremarkable.

Which of the following is the most likely diagnosis?

A) Conversion disorder.
B) Posterior fossa tumor
C) Viral labyrinthitis
D) Basilar type migraine
E) Familial hemiplegic migraine

299) Each of the following are recommendations to reduce the frequency and severity of migraine headaches *except.*

A) Regular sleep
B) Exercise
C) Elimination diets
D) Biofeedback
E) Stress management

300) You are caring for a 5 year old child who has been experiencing daily headaches over his left eye. He is not experiencing any nausea or vomiting, ataxia, visual or hearing deficits. He has been taking acetaminophen and ibuprofen several times a day with no relief. There is no evidence of head trauma. Other than a minor head trauma 6 weeks ago with no loss of consciousness there is no history of trauma.

The most likely cause of the chronic headaches would be:

A) Subdural hematoma
B) Epidural hematoma
C) Medication overuse headaches
D) Basilar type migraine
E) Familial hemiplegic migraine

301) You are caring for an 8 year old boy who was noted by the teachers to be periodically staring out the window without responding to her snapping her finger. Occasionally facial twitching occurs during these episodes. Which of the following would be the most appropriate treatment for this child?

A) Methylphenidate
B) Atomoxetine
C) Desipramine
D) Lamotrigine
E) Carbamazepine

302) Each of the following wold constitute appropriate treatment of infantile spasms *except*?

A) Ketogenic diet
B) Carbamazepine
C) Adrenocorticotropic hormone
D) Valproic acid
E) Topiramate

Nutrition

303) Each of the following statements regarding breast-feeding is true *Except*:

A) Human milk provides passive immunity via IgA
B) In general, pediatricians and other health care providers represent one of the major reasons for the increase in successful breast-feeding
C) Breast-feeding provides complete nutrition for growth, development, and hydration during the first 6 months of life
D) Family support is crucial for breast-feeding success

304) Breast milk is known to contain each of the following *EXCEPT* for:

A) IgA
B) Immunomodulating agents
C) IgG
D) Anti-inflammatory agents
E) Anti-microbial agents

305) Match each numbered description on the left to a vitamin <u>deficiency</u> on the right

1) Leading cause of blindness worldwide   (A) Phylloquinone
2) Hemolytic anemia   (B) Retinol
3) Hemorrhagic disease of the newborn   (C) Riboflavin
4) Peripheral paralysis and muscle weakness (D) Thiamine
5) Stomatitis and seborrheic dermatitis   (E) Tocopherol

306) Match each numbered item on the left to its corresponding <u>toxicity</u> on the right.

1) Liver toxicity   (A) Ascorbic acid
2) Vasodilator   (B) Niacin
3) Nephrocalcinosis   (C) Tocopherol

307) You have a moderately obese 16-year-old in your practice. Which of the following interventions for weight reduction would be the LEAST likely to be carried out successfully?

A) Exercise
B) Exercise with a peer
C) Reducing carbohydrates
D) Calorie reduction coordinated with the entire family
E) Long-term reduction of caloric intake

308) You are called to the nursery to evaluate a newborn that is 36 hours of age for persistent bilious vomiting. The MOST appropriate next step would be:

A) Have the child breast feed, and observe
B) Assess for overfeeding
C) Change to soy-based formula
D) Sepsis workup
E) Abdominal x-rays

309) Calciferol deficiency can result in each of the following EXCEPT:

A) High serum phosphatase levels
B) Infantile tetany
C) Poor growth
D) Pharyngeal ulcers
E) Osteomalacia

310) Niacin deficiency results in each of the following EXCEPT:

A) GI distress
B) Xerophthalmia
C) Dementia
D) Skin manifestations
E) Pellagra

311) A patient in your practice is diagnosed with celiac disease or gluten sensitivity enteropathy. You would be correct in suggesting that he avoid foods containing each of the following EXCEPT:

A) Wheat
B) Oats
C) Barley
D) Rye
E) Corn

312) You are evaluating a 9 month infant who has been increasingly fussy over the past 2 days. The family has recently returned from a trip aboard where the only available formula was evaporated milk which the child was fed exclusively on the trip. You examine the child and note that the child seems reluctant to being touched and prefers to sit in a frog position with hips and knees flexed. You also note some peripheral edema and swelling of the gums.

X-ray findings include ground glass appearance of the bones, thinning of the cortices, and calcified cartilage at the metaphysis.

The most appropriate treatment at this time would be:

A) Removal of the child from the home.
B) Avoidance of flies , since pathological tongue snagging of flies follows the preferred frog legged position
C) Calcium and vitamin D supplementation
D) Ascorbic acid supplementation
E) Fortified infant formula

313) You are evaluating a 4 year old boy presenting with increased irritability and headache over the past 3 days. Additional findings include some joint aches and lethargy. The child has not been experiencing nausea or vomiting and has remained afebrile. After 2 days of ibuprofen the headaches and irritability persist. Lumbar puncture reveals an elevated opening pressure with no red or white blood cells.

The most likely explanation for the physical findings would be:

A) Aseptic meningitis
B) Trauma
C) Retinol deficiency
D) Retinol toxicity
E) Migraine headaches

314) You are evaluating a dark skinned 12 month baby boy who as been exclusively breast fed up until now. The boy was born at 31 weeks gestation and was in the NICU for 1 week receiving supplemental oxygen for 3 days.

On physical exam the baby is below the 10ᵗʰ percentile for weight and height. You note some bowing of the legs and increased width of the wrists. Laboratory findings are significant for decreased serum calcium and phosphate with an elevated alkaline phosphatase level

A) Vitamin D deficiency
B) Vitamin E deficiency
C) Vitamin A deficiency
D) Iron deficiency anemia
E) Cystic fibrosis

315) Which of the following would be the most appropriate treatment of a child with mild dehydration who is tolerating clear fluids without emesis?

A) IV fluids and hospital admission
B) IV fluids , oral rehydration and discharge home on clear liquids for 24 hours
C) IV fluids, oral rehydration and discharge on diet of bananas, rice, apples, toast, and tea
D) Oral rehydration and discharge home on diet of bananas, rice , apples, toast and tea
E) Oral rehydration and discharge on a diet of vegetables, milk, meat and anything tolerated

316) You have admitted a 13 year old boy because of complications related Crohn's disease. You need to decide whether to provide nutrition with enteric formula via an NG tube or parenteral nutrition. The most important factor in making your decision would be:

A) The presence or absence of an anal fistula
B) The degree of inflammation noted on colonoscopy
C) The presence or absence of fever
D) The results of plain abdominal film
E) The presence or absence of digestive enzymes

317) **Which of the following is true regarding home prepared baby versus commercial baby food products in infants?**

A) Home prepared foods decreased the risk for development of food related allergies.
B) Honey can be added provided it has been properly stored
C) Home prepared products should be pureed and used immediately discarding any unused portions
D) Pureed home prepared foods can be frozen and used later
E) Standard bottled vegetables offer no advantage over bottled vegetables for infants

Pharmacology

318) **A teenager taking oral contraceptive pills should be concerned regarding its efficacy when taking which of the following herbal remedies?**

A) Valerian Root
B) Echinacea
C) Ginseng
D) Mooderall
E) St. John's Wort

319) **Which of the following herbal remedies is contraindicated in patients taking immunosuppressant medications?**

A) Echinacea
B) Ginseng
C) Sing Sing
D) St. John's Wort
E) Valerian Root

320) **Which of the following herbal remedies should type 2 diabetics taking oral hypoglycemic medications be concerned about?**

A) Echinacea
B) Ginseng
C) Valerian Root
D) St. John's Wort
E) Peppermint tea

321) **You are participating in a clinical trial. In fact, it is the "Clinical Trial of the Century" on Judge Joe Brown so you'd better get this question right or else Steve Colbert will be reviewing your pharmacological credentials on the Colbert Report. The medication is given twice a day and it reaches a steady state after 5 days. The half life of the drug is closest to:**

A) 12 hours
B) 24 hours
C) 36 hours
D) 72 hours
E) Who cares?

322) **Each of the following conditions can alter the serum level and, therefore, the therapeutic and toxicity of a variety of medications _EXCEPT_ for:**

A) Severe burns
B) Liver disease
C) Nephrotic syndrome
D) Hypertension
E) Juvenile polyps

Preventive

323) **Which of the following statements is true with regards to cholesterol levels in children?**

A) Screening for hypercholesterolemia should be started at age 1
B) In the absence of a positive family history for hypercholesteremia, screening will pick up an insignificant number of cases
C) An elevated HDL cholesterol level is a worrisome finding in children
D) Children older than 2-1/2 years of age should receive no more than 35% of their caloric intake from fat
E) Hypercholesteremia in children is due exclusively to diet and genetic predisposition.

324) **Hyperlipidemia can be found with each of the following conditions EXCEPT for:**
A) Sideroblastic anemia
B) Hyperthyroidism
C) Renal disease
D) Cushing syndrome
E) Hypothyroidism

325) **Intake of each of the following is associated with hyperlipidemia EXCEPT for:**
A) Isotretinoin
B) Ethanol
C) Methanol
D) Oral contraceptives
E) Steroid supplements

326) Which of the following is true regarding a 12 year old with a previous history of pertussis?

A) A previous diagnosis of pertussis is easy to confirm
B) Administering DTap to someone with a previous history of pertussis raises serious safety concerns
C) Administering Tdap to someone with a previous history of pertussis raises serious safety concerns
D) Tdap should be administered according to routine recommendations.
E) The duration protection after B pertussis infection is lifelong and no further immunization is indicated

327) An 8-year-old boy cut his hand on a broken bottle in the family garage. He received DTP immunization at 2, 4, and 6 months and DTaP at 15 months. Which of the following is the most appropriate tetanus vaccine regimen?

A) Pediatric strength diphtheria and tetanus toxoid
B) Adult strength diphtheria and tetanus toxoid
C) DTP
D) DTaP
E) No vaccine

328) The parents of a healthy 1-month-old female infant are concerned that he has colic because he is crying a lot. They note that his 4-year-old sibling had colic and that his father is "climbing the home entertainment center in frustration." Which of the following statements is TRUE regarding crying in infants?

A) As long as the infant-crying to father-whining ratio is less than 1:2 it is normal
B) Parental fear or anxiety plays a role in colic
C) Crying associated with flexion of the arms and legs is diagnostic of colic
D) Infants tend to cry more during the first month after birth
E) Newborn infants cry only in response to hunger

329) Of the following, the most significant problem associated with fatal accidents and injuries in adolescents is:

A) Depression
B) Ethanol consumption
C) Poor education on safety issues
D) Parental permissiveness
E) Dropping out of high school

330) In which of the following clinical situations is the live mumps vaccine contraindicated?

A) A child with ALL in remission who has not received chemotherapy for 5 months
B) A child with ITP who is receiving IV IG
C) A child with sickle cell disease
D) A child with stable HIV infection
E) A child with OM

331) Each of the following would be considered a contraindication for participation in contact sports EXCEPT:

A) Splenomegaly
B) Hepatomegaly
C) Acute diarrhea with dehydration
D) Impetigo
E) Unilateral testicle

332) Regarding suicide among adolescents, each of the following statements are true EXCEPT:

A) Suicide attempts are twice as frequent among females
B) The number of suicides completed is much higher among males
C) Suicide is the most common cause of death among adolescents
D) Only a fraction of adolescent suicide attempts come to medical attention
E) Firearms are the most prevalent method used in completed suicides

333) Which of the following would correlate best with *chronic alcohol abuse*?

A) Elevated serum gamma glutamyl transferase
B) Hypoglycemia
C) Metabolic acidosis
D) Decreased mean corpuscle volume
E) Elevated blood alcohol levels

334) Each of the following is true statements regarding drug abuse among adolescents EXCEPT:

A) Weapon carrying is associated with alcohol use
B) Fighting is more commonly seen with adolescents who use anabolic steroids
C) Teens who use anabolic steroids are at higher risk to abuse other drugs
D) Violent behavior is more common among adolescents who use drugs
E) Violent behavior is more common among male drug users than female drug users

Psychosocial

335) Which subgroup of teenagers is at the highest risk for suicide?

A) Those with mental retardation
B) Children of divorce
C) Homosexuals
D) Physically disabled
E) Those with chronic medical conditions

336) **Children with *mild* mental retardation are more likely to:**

A) Show delays in psychomotor skills in the first year of life
B) Have delayed speech and language abilities in the toddler years
C) Have a history of perinatal problems
D) Be diagnosed at school entry
E) Have a physical deformity associated with a syndrome

337) **While autism is largely understood to be an idiopathic disorder, it has been associated with each of the following conditions EXCEPT:**

A) Trisomy 21
B) Untreated phenylketonuria
C) Tuberous sclerosis
D) Fragile X syndrome
E) Anoxia during birth

338) **Regarding dyslexia, each of the following statements are true EXCEPT:**

A) It is frequently discovered in the fourth grade
B) It can go undetected into adulthood
C) It is an uncommon language disorder
D) There is evidence of a possible anatomical basis for the disorder
E) It tends to run in families

339) You are seeing a 3-year-old for a routine physical examination. The history and physical are all unremarkable. Developmental milestones are within normal limits, except for marked difficulty with speech. This is MOST suggestive of:

A) Infantile autism
B) Normal variation of language development
C) Hearing loss
D) Bilingual household
E) Lack of stimulation

340) Our next contestant on "Name That Age" is an infant who is able to babble and transfer a cube from one hand to another, yet drops one cube when handed another. He can crawl but does so by dragging his belly across the floor like a marine sneaking into enemy territory. These developmental milestones are MOST consistent with which age?

A) 5 months
B) 7 months
C) 9 months
D) 11 months
E) 18 years

341) The next contestant on Name That Age lifts his head and chest while lying down, coos, visually follows his mother around the room, and has a "primitive grasp". The MOST likely age is:

A) 1 month
B) 2 months
C) 4 months
D) 6 months
E) 9 months

342) **A couple who have recently adopted a newborn infant are there for the 2-week visit. They would like to know if and when the child should be told he was adopted. The BEST time to tell children of their adoption would be:**

A) When they bring it up themselves
B) If there are other siblings, it is best to avoid the topic
C) The age of 10, when they are mature enough to handle the information
D) When their verbal development allows for comprehension; around the age of 3 or 4 years
E) Never!

343) **A medication used for the treatment of ADHD that has recently fallen into disfavor is:**

A) Methylphenidate SR
B) Methylphenidate Short-acting
C) Dexedrine®
D) Amphetamine
E) Pemoline (Cylert®)

344) **A mother of a child in your practice cannot deny that her child is suffering from ADHD. However, she was referred to you because you are "open-minded" when it comes to treatment, and she wants to use "natural remedies" rather than the medications she has heard about that "turn kids into zombies" so lazy teachers do not have to do their jobs. Based on the latest findings your best approach would be to:**

A) Discuss the benefits of Kava Kava
B) Review the benefits of a trial of Valerian root and reinforcement of organizational skills and behavior
C) Review the child's diet for any preservatives, sugars, and dyes known to trigger ADHD, and speak with the teacher about seating arrangements
D) Discuss the benefits of a combination of herbs and supplements, including Kava Kava, Valerian root, Ginkgo biloba, and fish oil
E) Reassure her, evaluate her fears, and review what is known about methylphenidate and other medications to treat ADHD. Also discuss other non-medication methods to manage the condition, like behavior management

345) The parents of a 6-month-old girl consult you because the infant has been crying uncontrollably for the past 2 hours. Physical examination reveals an incarcerated inguinal hernia that you are able to reduce with some difficulty. You recommend that the hernia be repaired soon and explain the risk of recurrence of incarceration as well as the benefits and risks of surgery. The parents request that the surgery be delayed until the girl is at least one year of age. Of the following, your next step should be to:

A) Explore the parent's reasons for wishing to delay the surgery
B) Obtain a court order to proceed with surgery
C) Let the parents know if they ignore an incarcerated hernia they will be incarcerated
D) Refer the parents to another physician
E) Tell the parents that the risks of surgery are minimal

346) The parents of a 24-month-old boy are concerned because he displays *ritualistic behavior.* He has tantrums if he is interrupted, and he appears withdrawn. Which of the following is most likely to be associated with this child's problem?

A) Appropriate gesturing to indicate needs
B) Stranger anxiety
C) Abnormal language development
D) Hearing deficit
E) Maintenance of sustained eye contact

347) You are evaluating an infant who regards faces, smiles responsively, laughs, and occasionally stares at his hand for several seconds. He does not try to obtain a toy that is out of reach, or turn to the sound of a rattle. These findings are most consistent with a developmental age of:

A) 1 week
B) 2 months
C) 4 months
D) 6 months
E) 8 months

348) The parent of an 18-month-old girl consults you regarding the girl's language development. The girl has a 12-word vocabulary and uses a considerable amount of jargon, but she does not use any two-word phrases. Of the following, the best course of action at this time would be to:

A) Refer the girl for tympanometry
B) Refer the girl for brain stem evoked audiometry
C) Refer the girl to a speech pathologist
D) Refer the girl for a complete developmental evaluation
E) Assure the parent that language development is normal

349) You are giving a talk to a group of residents on the topic of homosexuality in teens. Which of the following would be true statements?

A) Sexual orientation and gender identity are synonymous
B) Sexual orientation is based solely on genetic predisposition
C) Homosexual teenagers are less likely to drop out of high school than their heterosexual peers
D) Sexual behavior and activity is a choice
E) Parents should be told that their children are free to choose their sexual orientation

350) A single mother brings her 7 year old daughter to be evaluated because she has found her in front of the television rubbing and touching her genitals on more than one occasion. The girl lives with mom but shares custody with her ex husband.

Which of the following additional behaviors would raise concern?

A) The girl's interest in wearing men's clothing
B) Vaginal discharge
C) Vaginal irritation
D) Imitation of adult sexual acts
E) Reluctance to undress in front of the mother

351) What would be the appropriate approach to a family with a child with a chronic, progressively debilitating illness that has kept the details away from them?

A) Continue to keep the information until it is too obvious to hide
B) Encourage them to explain the illness that is developmentally appropriate for age
C) Note that if they don't tell the child you will
D) Note that denying information from the child is akin to neglect requiring you to report them to the authorities
E) Offer to inform the child yourself in coordination with a therapist

352) Parents with vulnerable child syndrome have children with the following symptoms *except*:

A) Overachievement
B) Learning difficulties
C) Sleep difficulties
D) Risk behaviors that reinforce parental fears
E) Hyperactivity

353) Each of the following is true regarding "separation anxiety" disorder "except":

A) It is characterized by periods of exacerbation and remission
B) It occurs primarily in males
C) Symptoms can continue into adulthood
D) Peak onset is middle childhood
E) Children with separation anxiety disorder often have other psychiatric disorders

354) Resumption of school attendance after a time away from school is best performed by:

A) Having the parent stay in school for gradually decreased periods of time
B) Have the child initially attend on alternate days
C) A combination of home and school tutoring on alternating weeks
D) Immediate return without parent
E) Immediate return with liberal use of pharmacological agents

Pulmonary

355) Coughs, coughs, coughs—we see them all the time. Which one of the following statements regarding coughs in children is *TRUE*?

A) Coughs from an upper respiratory infection are most prominent during the day
B) Coughs due to pneumonia are most prominent at night, during naps, and the early morning.
C) The older a child is, the more likely a persistent cough is due to pneumonia.
D) Grunting is a common finding in infants with pneumonia
E) A persistent cough is a common presentation of pneumonia in the newborn period
F) The volume of coughing at symphony concerts is inversely proportional to the number of blackberries and cell phones that go off

356) A child receives general anesthesia for a hernia repair. What is the most common adverse reaction to isoflurane?

A) Hypothermia
B) Hyperthermia
C) Fluid overload
D) Hypokalemia
E) Hypernatremia
F) Hyponatremia

357) A previously healthy 18-month-old boy presents with sudden onset of cough for 2 days. The cough began while he was in the living room "The Wiggles" are on TV. He is afebrile with no sick contacts; Wheezing is heard over the right lower lobe. Of the following, the *most likely* diagnosis is:

A) An appropriate response to watching grown men prancing around pretending to be kids.
B) GE reflux
C) Asthma
D) Cystic fibrosis
E) foreign body aspiration

358) A 14-year-old asthmatic in your practice wants to play basketball and will be required to engage in strenuous training. The parents are concerned about exercise-induced asthma. Which of the following statements is the best advice to offer this family?

A) The boy should not participate in a strenuous sports program
B) Inhaled steroids should be administered prior to and after exercise
C) Steroid meter dose inhaler prior to strenuous exercise
D) Oxygen should be available on site
E) Beta-agonist bronchodilators rescue prior to strenuous exercise

359) A 15-month-old boy presents with a persistent cough of 2 weeks duration. The cough started suddenly while visiting his aunt. He has remained afebrile and has no history of asthma. The family history is negative for asthma and all other respiratory diseases. Physical examination is unremarkable except for cough. The chest x-ray report notes a right lower lobe hyperinflation and right upper lobe atelectasis. The *most likely* cause of the cough is:

A) Allergies to an environmental agent
B) Reactive airway disease
C) Psychogenic cough
D) Foreign body aspiration
E) Bronchiolitis

360) A 6-month-old infant is status post TE fistula repair and presents with wheezing and expiratory stridor. The MOST likely explanation would be:

A) Recurrence of TE fistula
B) Laryngomalacia
C) RSV bronchiolitis
D) Tracheomalacia
E) Lobar pneumonia

361) Each of the following is a risk factor for asthma persisting after adolescence EXCEPT:

A) Onset prior to 12 months
B) Recurrent viral illnesses
C) Elevated IgE levels
D) Eosinophilia
E) Rhinitis during the first year

362) Because of your dynamic personality, dapper clothing, and geometric taste in fine wine, you are called to speak to the local PTA on tuberculosis. They want to know the best way to tell if a child has TB. You CORRECTLY tell them:

A) Night sweats
B) Positive skin test
C) High fever
D) Fatigue
E) Painful cough

363) A 15-year-old boy with cystic fibrosis presents with rapid onset of severe respiratory distress and chest discomfort. He has been fully compliant with his daily regimen of antibiotics and other care. The symptoms can be best explained by:

A) Pseudomonas pneumonitis
B) Acute bronchospasm
C) Acute pneumothorax
D) Septic pleural effusion
E) Septic tank effusion
F) Acute pulmonary insufficiency

364) A 10-year-old girl has had a cough for the past 2 months. Findings on physical examination are normal except for a harsh, loud cough. Results of a CBC are normal. A CXR and sinuses x-rays are normal. Peak expiratory flow rates are normal before and after exercise. A tic disorder is suspected of being the underlying cause. Which of the following would best support the tentative diagnosis?

A) Control of cough with albuterol therapy
B) A family history of a tic disorder
C) Persistence of cough after administration of codeine
D) Absence of cough during sleep
E) A positive response to phenothiazine therapy

365) A 14-year-old old boy has had a recurrent cough associated with exercise for the past 6 months. The cough is episodic but has been worse since he joined the cross-country team. He reports occasional whitish mucoid sputum. His medical history and results of a review of systems are unremarkable. Physical findings are normal. Which of the following is *most likely* to yield the correct diagnosis?

A) X-ray study of chest
B) Direct laryngoscopy
C) Blood eosinophil
D) Serum IgE concentration
E) Pulmonary function test

366) Which one of the following statements is true regarding the management of acute asthma exacerbations in children?

A) Inhaled anticholinergics should be routinely used in cases of severe asthma exacerbations
B) If a patient presents with fever and a cough during an acute exacerbation they should be routinely started on antibiotics
C) A chest x-ray is helpful in all children experiencing an acute asthma exacerbation
D) Steroids improve pulmonary function compared with the use of bronchodilators alone with acute asthma
E) Short course of steroids are of equal efficacy as longer course requiring tapering in all cases

367) Which of the following describes a patient with *mild persistent* asthma?

A) General symptoms greater than 2 times a week and night symptoms greater than 2 times a month
B) General symptoms and night symptoms greater than 2 times a week
C) General symptoms and night symptoms greater than 2 times a month
D) General symptoms greater than 2 times a month and night symptoms greater than 2 times a week
E) General and night symptoms greater than 2 times a month

368) Each of the following is true regarding the chronic management of children with asthma *except?*

A) Chronic use of inhaled steroids has a minimal impact on adult height if any
B) The impact of inhaled steroids on growth can be minimized with the use of spacers and mouth rinsing after use
C) Chest x-rays in preschool children can be useful during acute exacerbations
D) Pulmonary function testing is the most objective measurement of improvement for preschool children
E) Children whose asthma is triggered only by viral illness have moderate persistent asthma

369) Which of the following are true regarding the epidemiology and risk factors associated with asthma?

A) African American and Caucasian children are hospitalized with equal frequency
B) Early child care exposure with frequent viral infections increases the risk for persistent asthma at age 7
C) Younger siblings in a given household have a higher incidence of allergies and asthma
D) Children in child care have a higher incidence of wheezing before age 2
E) Children in child care have a lower incidence of wheezing before age 2

370)   Each of the following statements are true regarding pneumonia in children *except:*

A) It's incidence is higher in children from lower socioeconomic levels
B) Boys have a higher incidence of pneumonia than girls
C) Fever and cough are the hallmark symptoms
D) Chest x-ray confirmation is needed before treatment with antibiotics
E) Tachypnea may not be a presenting sign.

Renal

371)   The mother of a 15-year-old has hypertension and has just been diagnosed with *autosomal-dominant kidney disease.* The child is asymptomatic. Physical findings and urine analysis are normal. Which of the following is the MOST appropriate next step in the evaluation of this child?

A) MRI
B) Renal US
C) Repeat urinalysis and serum calcium levels
D) Magnetic angiography (MRA)
E) Urine creatinine clearance study

372)   A 13-year-old boy is being followed for microscopic hematuria noted on several occasions over the past year. His history is negative and the family history reveals no evidence of renal disease or hematuria. His urinalysis shows 30 RBC/hpf and is negative for protein. Erythrocyte casts are noted. Serum creatinine and C3 are both normal. The urine calcium creatinine ratio as well as abdominal U/S are normal. Which of the following is the MOST appropriate next step?

A) Voiding cystourethrogram
B) Repeat the urine analysis in followup
C) Renal biopsy
D) IVP
E) Abdominal CT

373) **Each of the following renal diseases can result in hypertension EXCEPT:**

A) Bartter's syndrome
B) Pyelonephritis
C) Glomerulonephritis
D) Williams syndrome
E) Neurofibromatosis

374) **Each of the following diseases can affect the kidney's ability to concentrate urine EXCEPT:**

A) Sickle cell disease
B) Acute tubular necrosis
C) Diabetes insipidus
D) Barters syndrome
E) Post strep glomerulonephritis

375) **During a routine physical exam you note the following results on a urinalysis.**

Specific gravity of 1.023, pH of 5.5, Protein 2 $^+$, negative for blood, WBC 0-4, RBC 0-3, epithelial cells 3-5, and bacteria – few. The history and physical exam are unremarkable. The MOST appropriate next step would be:

A) Obtain a renal ultrasound
B) Obtain a first AM urine protein/creatinine ratio
C) Obtain serum BUN, creatinine, liver function tests, and serum albumin
D) Urine culture and presumptive treatment with trimethoprim-sulfamethoxazole
E) Obtain a 24-hour urine protein

376) **Low serum C_3 levels are seen with each of the following EXCEPT:**

A) Focal segmental glomerulonephritis
B) Membranoproliferative glomerulonephritis
C) Acute post strep glomerulonephritis
D) Lupus nephritis

377) You are evaluating a 6-year-old child for nocturnal enuresis. Before dismissing it as idiopathic, you would be justified in ruling out each of the following EXCEPT:

A) Diabetes insipidus
B) Sickle cell disease
C) Seizure
D) SIADH
E) Lumbosacral anomaly

378) Each of the following is a true statement regarding hemolytic uremic syndrome EXCEPT:

A) It occurs primarily during the summer months
B) It affects primarily pre-schoolers
C) Has a predilection for families of lower socioeconomic status
D) Has a predilection for families of higher socioeconomic status
E) Occurs more commonly in the Northern US and Canada

379) Which of the following types of renal stones form only in the setting of infection?

A) Calcium oxalate
B) Struvite
C) Uric acid
D) Cystine
E) Rolling

380) A child with inflammatory bowel disease develops a renal stone. Which of the following stone would be most likely?

A) Oxalate
B) Struvite
C) Uric Acid
D) Cystine
E) Mick Jagger

381) Which of the following constitute first line therapy for patients with hematuria and renal stones due to hypercalciuria?

A) Thiazide diuretics
B) Increase water intake
C) Low sodium diet
D) Alkalinization of urine
E) B and C

382) In addition to hematuria which of the following additional findings would raise the concern for a progressive renal disease?

A) Red cast cells
B) White blood cells
C) Proteinuria
D) Abdominal pain
E) Fever

383) Each of the following is consistent with congenital nephrotic syndrome except:

A) Small kidneys on renal ultrasound
B) Anasarca
C) Low serum thyroid –binding globulin
D) Low serum transferrin
E) Hyperechogenic renal cortex

384) You are evaluating a 4 year old with mild proteinuria. She has had a fever of 101.2 over the past 3 days. Her white blood cell count and hematocrit and hemoglobin are within normal limits

The most appropriate management at this time would be:

A) Renal ultrasound
B) Renal biopsy
C) 24 hour urine creatinine collection
D) One time measure of urine creatinine
E) Repeat urine analysis in 3 weeks

385) Each of the following is an adverse effect of ACE inhibitors in children *except* for

A) Hypokalemia
B) Neutropenia
C) Angioedema
D) Dry cough
E) Anemia

Rheumatology

386) All of the following are considered major Jones criteria *EXCEPT* for:

A) Arthralgia and erythema chronicum migrans
B) Carditis
C) Arthritis and erythema marginatum
D) Chorea
E) Subcutaneous nodules

387) **All of the following are true with regards to Kawasaki disease** *EXCEPT:*

A) It is more common among Asian populations
B) It is more common among girls
C) It is more prevalent in the winter and spring than in the summer and fall
D) Most cases occur in children between 4 –5 years of age
E) IV gamma globulin given in the acute phase reduces the risk for coronary artery disease

388) **All of the following are associated with Henoch Schönlein purpura** *EXCEPT* **for:**

A) IgA nephropathy
B) Proteinuria
C) Hematuria
D) Thrombocytopenia
E) Anaphylactoid purpura

389) **An 8 year old boy reports to your office complaining of 2 weeks of lethargy and just not feeling like playing with the other kids. He has had a low-grade fever which t responds to Tylenol, but only for four hours and then his parents have to give him another dose.**

On physical exam you see that his throat is non-injected, TM is clear, and there is no nasal discharge. Lungs are clear, and you note a systolic ejection click heard best at the apex. Abdominal exam reveals a non-tender abdomen, soft with no guarding or rebound, no hepatomegaly but 2 – 3 cm. splenomegaly. No significant joint aches; however, you do note some tenderness over the pads of his fingers. The best study to confirm this diagnosis would be:

A) Abdominal CT and serological studies
B) Bone scan
C) Blood culture
D) Cardiac echo and chest X ray
E) IV Ig based on your presumptive diagnosis, with close follow-up of signs of coronary arterial dilation

390) Each of the following would be suggestive of a new case of rheumatic fever EXCEPT:

A) Nonspecific pink macules that cover the trunk, prolonged PR interval, arthralgia, and a positive throat culture for group A beta hemolytic strep
B) A marked deterioration in their handwriting, motional lability
C) Firm, non-tender, pea-sized nodules on knees and elbows and over the spine
D) Pericardial effusion, with first-degree heart block
E) High, spiking fever for 6 days, bilateral conjunctivitis, skin peeling noted on the skin of the fingers

391) Each of the following is a clinical manifestation of Kawasaki disease EXCEPT:

A) Thrombocytosis
B) Bacterial meningitis
C) Sterile pyuria
D) Hydrops of the gallbladder
E) Conjunctivitis

392) Which one of the following is associated with systemic lupus erythematosus?

A) Conjunctivitis
B) Erythema chronicum migrans
C) Erythema multiforme
D) Palmar erythema
E) Erythema marginatum

393) In patients with systemic lupus erythematosus which organ system is likely to cause the most serious morbidity and mortality?

A) Hematological
B) Central nervous system
C) Renal
D) Cardiac
E) It is too variable to determine

394) Which one of the following maternal serum antibodies is most associated with congenital heart block in a newborn?

A) ANA
B) Anti –Sm. (Smith)
C) Anti-ds DNA
D) Anti-Ro
E) Anti-La

395) Which of the following is true regarding the epidemiology of systemic lupus erythematosus?

A) African –Americans are the most susceptible racial group to develop lupus
B) Only 5% of all patients who have lupus are diagnosed in childhood
C) After puberty the female to male ratio drops down to 2:1
D) Prior to puberty the female to male ratio is 3:1
E) Most pediatric patients are diagnosed prior to puberty

Substance Abuse

396) Which one of the following statements with regards to amphetamine and methamphetamine is *TRUE*?

A) The N-methyl group on methamphetamine results in decreased peripheral side effects
B) Amphetamines work by decreasing presynaptic uptake
C) D-form and L-form are equal pharmacokinetically
D) Phentolamine and nifedipine are used in acute overdose situations
E) Haloperidol is used to treat the aggression/agitation that often accompanies amphetamine abuse

397) You are working as a camp doctor primarily to relax and get free tuition for your kid. You are reeling in a small mouth bass, when you are awoken by the hum of an approaching panic stricken crowd. Apparently it is 9AM and you were only dreaming about fishing.

They bring in a 12 year old boy believed to be drunk. He was found in the woods near his bunk, laughing ataxic, slurring his words. Fortunately you have a drug test which is negative for alcohol, Cannibis and all drugs on the panel.

You observe the boy for an hour and the symptoms quickly resolve over 30 minutes

The most likely diagnosis explanation for the clinical presentation would be:

A) Lab error
B) Glue inhalation
C) Malingering behavior
D) Poison mushroom ingestion
E) Poppy Seed toxicity

398) Sudden death from cocaine toxicity would most likely be due to

A) Trauma secondary to inappropriate behavior
B) Cardiac arrhythmias
C) Barotrauma following Valsalva maneuver to increase inhalation
D) Cerebral vascular accident secondary to hypertension
E) Bilateral pneumothoraces

399) You are evaluating a teenager in the emergency room who is sleepy. Pupils are equal and normal sized but react sluggishly to light. The conjunctiva are not injected

Which of the following substances could account for these clinical findings?

A) Alprazolam
B) Amphetamine
C) Phencyclidine
D) Heroin
E) Marijuana

400) You are evaluating a teenager who while playing football, suddenly collapses on the field. You evaluate him and he is disoriented to time and place and is tachycardic, tachypneic and has a recorded fever of 104.5 His pupils are equal, reactive and normal size.

Which of the following would be most appropriate in treating this patient once his airway and breathing have been established?

A) Provide him with a cool glass of water
B) Rapid cooling to 101.8F but no lower
C) Rapid cooling to 98.6
D) Naloxone
E) IV dextrose rapid infusion

Answers

Adolescent

1)   E)   This is one of the rare cases where crossing out an answer with the word *all* would not be a good move. Gynecomastia occurs in up to 50% of adolescent boys and while marijuana use is considered a risk factor it is not *rare* among non marijuana users. However, since all of the other answers are not correct the process of elimination would leave you no choice.

2)   C)   Breast development consisting of glandular tissue beyond the areolae with no secondary mounding of the nipples or areolae is a description of a sexual maturity rating of 3 for breast development.

3)   D)   The history is most consistent with *non-specific vaginitis.* Eighty percent of prepubertal vaginitis results in negative bacterial and fungal cultures. A history should be taken to assess for the use of bubble bath which can cause vaginal irritation. Sitz baths and perhaps looser fitting clothing will often solve the problem; therefore, reassurance that the discharge is normal is the most appropriate management.

4)   D)   Osteogenic sarcoma often presents in active adolescents, and is first diagnosed incidentally after pain that persists after an injury and is out of proportion to the level of trauma incurred. The initial symptoms are often mistakenly attributed to pain secondary to a sports injury. However, this child exhibits none of the other signs of osteogenic sarcoma. He has been previously well.

      Normal lab values can also be seen with osteogenic sarcoma; however, one would expect to find elevated alkaline phosphatase and lactic dehydrogenase levels, both of which are within normal range.

      Osteoid osteoma usually presents as pain at night relieved by ibuprofen, and there is nothing in the history to suggest this as the cause of the pain.

      The HCT has dropped slightly, which could be attributed to the bleeding into the hematoma. Therefore the most likely diagnosis is a deep tissue hematoma.

5)   E) Pour a tub of Gatorade over them and ask "Cool enough for you guys?" Providing unrestricted access to fluids is the best way to prevent heat-related illnesses.

6)   E) Most cases of endocervical chlamydia infection in females are asymptomatic (70% or more) It is also not possible to base the diagnosis on physical exam alone since physical exam is usually unremarkable. Urethritis secondary to chlamydia infection is characterized by sterile pyuria.

Fitz Hugh Curtis which manifests as right upper quadrant tenderness is due to *peri*hepatitis not hepatitis. Endometriosis is also a possible complication of chlamydia infection in adolescent females.

7)   C) The question clearly states that the reason for the symptoms is a recurrent chlamydia urethritis so gonococcal urethritis would not be the explanation. Azithromycin should be adequate treatment so a broader spectrum antibiotic isn't necessary. There is nothing to suggest poor compliance with one treatment. However nothing is stated regarding his partner being treated as well, therefore the most likely explanation is reinfection by his untreated partner who is there now and can be evaluated and treated as well.

8)   C) An easy mnemonic to calculate the ideal body weight for females in questions involving the possibility of an eating disorder is 100 pounds for 60 inches in height plus 5 pounds for each additional inch.

For males the formula is 106 pounds for 60 inches plus 6 pounds for each additional inch.

9)   A) Severe bradycardia, hypotension especially with orthostatic changes and arrhythmias especially a prolonged QT interval on EKG are all indications for hospital admission in a patient with anorexia nervosa. Tachycardia in an otherwise stable patient would not be an indication for hospital admission.

10) C) The patient in this vignette is experiencing moderate bleeding Moderate bleeding consists of cycles lasting less than 3 weeks (as in this scenario) or menses lasting more than 7 days. In addition the hemoglobin is greater than 10 (again as in this scenario)

Treatment of moderate dysfunctional uterine bleeding consists of oral contraceptive pills and close followup including serial hematocrits. Iron supplements and maintenance of a menstrual calendar would be appropriate in any adolescent female even those not experiencing dysfunctional uterine bleeding.

A packed red cell transfusion would not be indicated in a clinically stable patient experiencing moderate dysfunctional uterine bleeding.

Allergy & Immunology

11)
1) (C) Adenosine deaminase deficiency.
2) (A) **B**ruton's disease primarily affects **B** cells.
3) (B) T and B cells counts are normal. In common variable immunodeficiency, both T and B cell counts are affected, but it is transient and, therefore, most of the time these patients have normal T and B cell counts.
4) (D) Since Di George's syndrome is associated with the absence of parathyroid tissue, there is no parathyroid hormone, decreased vitamin D, and therefore lowered serum calcium resulting in hypocalcemia. Di George's syndrome is also associated with little or no thymus, resulting in decreased T cell counts.
5) (E) Elevated immunoglobulins. During the first year of life a child with HIV can have elevated immunoglobulin levels. However, these are mostly non-functional immunoglobulins, essentially soldiers AWOL (Absent without Leave).
6) (C) Adenosine deaminase deficiency. It is the disorder that the "Bubble Boy" in *Seinfeld* had, and an easy way to remember this is "yADA, yADA, yADA"— the phrase made famous on the show is associated with ADA deficiency and severe combined immunodeficiency.

12)   E)   Deficiencies of complement components are associated with an increased risk for recurrent encapsulated organisms such as with pneumococcemia, meningococcemia, and gonococcemia.

13)   E)   Children with deficiency of C6 are at risk for both *Neisseria meningococcus* and *Neisseria gonococcus*. Easy to remember if you change it to "Nice 6 area".

14)   D)   This is a "late food reaction" and therefore a *non-IgE* mediated reaction to the cow milk protein. In this case the infant was probably already sensitized to cow milk protein and is experiencing an anaphylactic reaction. Skin testing will therefore be negative.

15)   E)   When you see the words **eczema along with thrombocytopenia**, think Wiskott-Aldrich syndrome.

While *Pneumocystis carinii* pneumonia is commonly seen with AIDS, the normal serum immunoglobulins coupled with eczema and thrombocytopenia makes AIDS less likely. In fact, serum immunoglobulins would usually be elevated in AIDS.

16)   D)   When you are presented with a child with recurrent infections you should first consider an immunodeficiency as the underlying cause. If you are given the additional information of bruising easily and eczema Wiskott Aldrich Syndrome should jump out at you.

17)   A)   Ataxia telangiectasia presents in early childhood with regression of motor milestones. Recurrent sinopulmonary infections involving encapsulated organism is seen in ataxia telangiectasia.

Immunologic findings include decreased IgA levels as well as decreased IgG levels and T-lymphocyte deficiency.

Ataxia telangiectasia is inherited in an autosomal *recessive* pattern.

18)   A)   The most frequent form of chronic granulomatous disease (CGD) is inherited in an x-liked recessive pattern. However the other forms are inherited in an autosomal recessive pattern.

In addition to the nitroblue tetrazolium test, it can also be diagnosed by demonstrating defective oxidase activity in granulocytes via the dihydrorhodamine flow cytometry test.

Urinary retention and bowel obstruction are potential complications.

Prophylactic treatment is indicated with trimethoprim/sulfamethoxazole and itraconazole. Subcutaneous interferon-gamma therapy is also used.

19)   E)   Even though theophylline is rarely used to treat asthma anymore, you are still expected to know its pharmakinetics on the exam.

Both phenobarbital and rifampin increase theophylline clearance in the liver and therefore would reduce theophylline levels.

Cimetidine would lead to elevated theophylline levels and ranitidine would have no effect.

20)   D)   Oral diphenhydramine and corticosteroids can be used as adjunct treatment. However the most appropriate treatment of an acute anaphylactic reaction is epinephrine (1:1000) SQ 0.01 mg/kg.

The steroids are used to prevent a phase II reaction a few hours after the initial reaction.

Cardiology

21)   D)   Each of the items listed are common causes of non-cardiac chest pain in children except foreign body aspiration, which typically causes unilateral wheezing and acute onset of persistent coughing in a toddler.

Note that on the exam they will not describe any suspicion of FB aspiration other than an acute onset of coughing in a crawling infant or toddler.

22)   1)   C
       2)   B
       3)   A

A **left axis deviation** can be seen with AV canal defects, tricuspid atresia, double outlet right ventricle, and sometimes with a normal heart. With a hypertrophic cardiomyopathy one would have an increased left ventricular mass; however, *one would not expect to see a left axis deviation on EKG.*

With right ventricular hypertrophy one would expect to see *right axis deviation.* This would be the case with tetralogy of Fallot, pulmonary stenosis, or transposition of the great vessels.

23)   1) B
     2) A
     3) C

The **Still's murmur** is due to harmonic vibrations of the left ventricular outflow tract therefore it is **low in pitch and often musical in quality** Of course one man's music is another man's shrilling noise however you only need to know the description on the exam They won't be playing an MP3 file for you.

The **pulmonary flow murmur** is a **systolic ejection-type murmur** *that is higher in pitch than Still's murmur* and is **heard best over the upper left sternal border**. It is caused by normal turbulence across the right ventricular outflow tract and pulmonary valve.

The **cervical venous hum** is caused by the normal, turbulent flow patterns at the junction of the innominate vein drainage into the superior vena cava. It is often **present only when sitting or standing.**

24)   A)   *Paroxysmal hypercyanotic attacks* which are also known as *Tet spells* are a particular problem during the first 2 years of life. The infant becomes hyperpneic and restless, cyanosis increases, gasping respirations ensue, and syncope may follow.

Management would include
1) Placement of the infant on the abdomen in the knee-chest position, making certain that there is no constricting clothing;
(2) Administration of oxygen (although increasing inspired oxygen will not reverse cyanosis due to intracardiac shunting);
(3) Injection of morphine subcutaneously in a dose not in excess of 0.2 mg/kg.

25)   E)   Since this child is exhibiting signs of **dig toxicity,** it would be most appropriate to reduce the current dose.

Therefore the question is really asking "When do you obtain a dig level after reducing the dose?

The most meaningful level would be obtained at least a week after changing the dose.

Likewise the best time to obtain a dig level after starting treatment would be at least one week after starting treatment.

26)   E)   Despite the normal physical exam which would imply a normal neurological exam this scenario is consistent with a thromboembolus that has dislodged into cerebral circulation. Therefore, a head CT would be the most appropriate next diagnostic step.

27)   D)   The key here is the word "small". A patient with a **small VSD** has a relatively benign lesion that is amenable to a "normal life". This can be described as a *loud, harsh or blowing; holosystolic murmur heard best over the lower left sternal border and can be accompanied by a thrill.*[1]

While these patients may be at risk for pulmonary hypertension, this can be screened by EKG.

It is also important to note that under the new SBE prophylaxis guidelines patients with VSDs are not given prophylactic antibiotics before surgical procedures.

Overall, patients with VSD do lead a normal life with no limitations when it comes to sports and physical activity.

28)   E)   Captopril reduces ventricular afterload by decreasing vascular resistance.[2] Another example of a medication that serves as an "afterload" reducing agent is *hydralazine.*

Digoxin enhances cardiac contractility.
Furosemide, **spironolactone**, and **chlorothiazide** are all diuretics.
  · *Furosemide (Lasix®)* inhibits the reabsorption of sodium and chloride in the distal tubules and the loop of Henle.
  · *Chlorothiazide* affects reabsorption of electrolytes in the renal tubules and requires potassium supplementation when given.
  · *Spironolactone* inhibits aldosterone production and enhances potassium retention. It is often given with chlorothiazide instead of potassium supplements.

29)   B)   A syncopal episode that occurs during exercise must be worked up for a cardiac cause, especially **prolonged QT syndrome,** which can result in sudden death if not diagnosed and managed.

Often there can be a family history of "unexplained" sudden death in a young person.

Treatment is via **beta-adrenergic drugs** and sometimes **cardiac pacemaker** placement.

---

[1] Not unlike the one you will experience when you get the question right.
[2] If you must know, it does so by inhibiting angiotensin-converting enzyme, thus blocking the production of angiotensin II.

30) A) This cardiac cath is consistent with a normal heart. Blood coming across the RA, RV into the PA is desaturated blood on the way to the lungs with a low pressure gradient from the RV to the pulmonary artery.

On the left side the blood returns from the lungs saturated and the pressure gradient across the aorta is akin to systemic blood pressure.

31) E) This is a cardiac cath consistent with transposition of the great vessels. The key to answering this correctly is the reversal of the pressure seen in the respective ventricles and the gradients across the pulmonary artery and aorta.

They are reversed or *transpositioned* once you identify this difference this question becomes a slam dunk

32) C) The key to recognizing this cardiac catheterization as **pulmonary stenosis** is the markedly decreased pressure gradient in the pulmonary artery and the slightly increased pressure gradient in the right ventricle.

33) C) In this cardiac catheterization you will have to identify the increased right ventricle pressure along with slightly increased saturation of the RV and pulmonary artery. This would be due to mixing of oxygenated blood which could only come about by left to right shunting. Given the combination of increased right ventricular pressure and increased saturation, this could best be explained by blood flow from the left side to the RV, across a VSD.

34) E) In this cardiac catheterization there is no change in the oxygen saturations. The only change is the increased pressure in the left ventricle and the decreased pressure in the aorta. This is consistent with an increased pressure gradient due to **aortic stenosis.**

35) E) While cholecystitis can present with RUQ tenderness with radiation to the shoulder the unremarkable abdominal exam in this patient rules this out. There is no evidence for GERD causing the chest pain and the lack of pain with tactile pressure makes costochondritis unlikely and therefore ibuprofen would not be indicated.

Given the description of the child's 45 year old father being on a medication to reduce his blood pressure there is a very good chance the father has familial hypercholesterolemia. As such the chest pain the patient is experiencing may very well be angina requiring a cardiology referral and restriction of all strenuous activity until cleared.

This is one of the rare instances where referring to a specialist would be appropriate.

36) D) Of all the choices listed only cyanosis distinguishes a simple atrioseptal defect from total anomalous venous return.

Cognition, Language & Learning

37) B) Remember age 2 (2/4 = 50 % intelligible), age 3 (3/4 = 75% intelligible), age 4 (4/4 = 100% intelligible). You might be tempted to choose D, but you probably haven't had a lengthy conversation with an 18 year old lately.

38) D) Since defects in vision, hearing and/or language can have devastating effects on a child's development, identifying these problems **early** is the most effective way to identify and intervene and/or prevent developmental disabilities.

39)   C)   This is a classic description of fragile X syndrome and a karyotype test would be the simplest one to order to rule it out (or in).

40)   A)   They become eligible at age 18 regardless of the parents need. At age 18 financial eligibility for medicaid and social security benefits no longer depend on the income of the parents. The need is based on the income of the "adult" with mental retardation Eligibility continues throughout adulthood based on the ability or inability to support themselves.

41)   D)   Behavioral management strategies are the key element in *Individual Education Plans* (IEP)

While anticonvulsants to treat irritability and mood swings (not seizures) and Alpha-2-adrenergic agents to control aggression and self-injurious behaviors are a part of IEPs they are not considered to be the key element

Likewise tutoring and vocational training are a part of IEPs but they are not considered to be the key component.

Critical Care

42)   C)   The formula is 7 ml/kg and therefore 100ml is the closest. I believe 6 trillion would be the correct answer if you were asked to calculate the number of people who vote more than once on American Idol, but this is of course beyond the scope of this book.

43)   D)   Botulism toxin acts by blocking the release of acetylcholine from the presynaptic neuron.

44) D) Prompt CPR including mouth to mouth resuscitation coupled with chest compressions can prove to be life saving and is the most important step to take immediately after a child is rescued from a near drowning episode.

Attempts to clear the airway including the Heimlich maneuver are not helpful and may prove to be more harmful by inducing emesis instead.

45) B) Noncardiogenic pulmonary edema, impaired oxygenation, bilateral pulmonary infiltrates is the diagnostic triad of ARDS. However the clinical manifestations can consist of tachypnea, diminished lung compliance, increasing hypoxemia which ultimately results in respiratory failure secondary to muscle fatigue.

ARDS usually occurs soon after lung injury secondary to drowning, however it can occur hours and even days after initial lung injury.

ARDS is due to *alveolar capillary insult resulting in increased pulmonary capillary permeability.*

In addition to drowning RDS can be secondary to:

· Pneumonia
· Aspiration
· Lung contusion
· Smoke inhalation
· Blood product transfusion
· Sepsis

46) D) A child with Reye syndrome who is unresponsive for 12 hours does not meet the clinical criteria for brain death since you would also need to have a known irreversible cause. A flat line EEG would be consistent with brain death but not pathognomic, especially if the neurologists are considered to be brain dead by their non-neurologist colleagues.

An irreversible cause with complete absence of brainstem function for 12 hours would be among the clinical criteria for brain death but in and of itself would not be pathognomic

Of the choices listed the only one which is pathognomic for brain death would be the absence of blood flow to intracranial arteries confirmed with cerebral nucleotide study.

Dermatology

47) B) While erythema marginatum is a rare manifestation of rheumatic fever, of all the rashes listed it is most associated with rheumatic fever. It is also one of the 5 major Jones criteria. It is a transient red macule that spreads and is characterized by central clearing.

48) D) Flashlamp-pumped, pulsed dye laser is the safest and most effective treatment for a port-wine stain on the face. It avoids thermal injury to the surrounding tissue. The appearance of the skin is then normal, with no scarring. Treatment can even begin during infancy. The other correct choice would have been "tunable dye laser therapy". Dermablend® is a form of "cosmetic" masking, which is essentially makeup; it would clearly not be the "most" effective method. Contralateral tattooing would probably raise eyebrows in the plastic surgery community and perhaps even in the tattooing community.

49) 1) (D) - Erythema multiforme
   2) (C) - Erythema infectiosum, whose nom de guerre is 5th disease.
   3) (E) - Erythema migrans
   4) (B) - Erythema nodosum
   5) (F) - Erythema confusiosum. It *is* difficult to keep these straight, isn't it.
   6) (A) - Erythema marginatum.

Erythema multiforme's involving the mucous membranes is an important component to making the correct diagnosis.

Erythema infectiosum is the formal name of Fifths disease which is caused by parvovirus B 19.

Erythema chronicum migrans is the rash seen in 70% of cases of Lyme disease.

Erythema nodosum is associated with inflammatory bowel disease.

Erythema confusiosum is what you are experiencing right now, which is eyes glazed over trying to determine which erythema is correct on the Exam-ema.

Erythema marginatum is erythematous macules on the back associated with rheumatoid arthritis.

50)   C)   While erythema nodosum is not unique to tuberculosis, of all the rashes listed erythema nodosum is the only one associated with tuberculosis. Erythema nodosum is characterized by tense, painful nodules found on the skin over the tibia. These nodules are usually purple in color. They can also be seen in inflammatory bowel disease and several other infections, including strep and fungal disease.

51)   E)   While periungual fibromas and café au lait spots can be seen in tuberous sclerosis, they are not seen as consistently as ash leaf macules. Ash leaf macules are seen in 90% of the cases. Again, reading the question carefully would be critical here.

For those of you who do not frequent mountain terrain and are unfamiliar with what the leaf of an ash tree looks like, the image to the right is what we came up with. Your best bet is to look this up in an atlas. It is basically a well-demarcated area of hypopigmentation.

Other cutaneous lesions associated with tuberous sclerosis include **facial angiofibromas,** which are fleshy growths seen around the nose or cheeks. It is a classic image tested in the picture section of the certification exam. Another lesion is the **shagreen patch.** It is typically described as a roughened raised lesion with an orange peel consistency,[3] seen above the belt line or the lumbosacral area.

52)   D)   *Borrelia burgdorferi* is the tick-borne spirochete that causes Lyme disease. The typical rash seen in Lyme disease is *erythema migrans,* a circular rash that is clear in the middle. In most cases, it develops within 30 days of the tick bite.

53)   A)   The rash described is seborrheic dermatitis. It typically appears during the first two months of life. It can also appear on the scalp, cheeks, and forehead. It requires no intervention and will resolve over several weeks. Therefore, parental reassurance is the correct answer.

Of course in the clinical world pediatricians frequently might treat mild cases with Nizoral shampoo, and possibly a mild topical steroid. However for purposes of the exam mild seborrheic dermatitis in a 6 week old would not require intervention.

---

[3] The origin of this word is for "shagreen leather" which has an orange peel texture. It would make more sense to call it an orange peel patch, since there are probably only two doctors out there who have actually heard of shagreen leather.

54) B) This rash is due to zinc deficiency. The tip-off should be that the infant is a former premie. Premature babies are at risk for zinc deficiency due to high requirements, decreased zinc stores, and inadequate zinc in hyperalimentation nutrition.

In addition to the typical rash, zinc deficiency also results in irritability and diarrhea. Another disorder worth noting is "*acrodermatitis enteropathica*", which is an autosomal recessive disorder that results in the impaired GI absorption of zinc. Manifestations include dermatitis, diarrhea, and alopecia.

55) 1) (C)
2) (B)
3) (E)
4) (A)
5) (D)

Tinea capitis, which is a highly contagious fungal infection of the scalp (ringworm of the scalp), can manifest with inflammation and black dots. The black dots are actual stubs of broken hairs.

Alopecia totalis is, of course, Latin for "total hair loss", and this would include the loss of eyebrow hair.

Trichotillomania is caused by compulsive pulling and/or twisting of the hair until it breaks off, resulting in incomplete patches of hair loss and the resulting *moth-eaten appearance.*

Alopecia areata is characterized by the complete loss of hair within well-defined round patches and is of a non-infectious etiology. Although unconfirmed, it is felt to be an autoimmune disorder.

Alopecia neurotica is the total, partial, or incomplete hair loss resulting from the stress of preparing for the board exam; *sometimes* the hair returns. When the hair *does* return, the volume that returns is directly proportional to the exam score; there is no other cure.

56) C) This is most likely post-*Strep* glomerulonephritis secondary to a cutaneous infection due to a nephritogenic strain of *Strep*. The U/A will help establish the diagnosis by the presence of RBCs and RBC casts. Unlike rheumatic fever, the evidence that antibiotics will affect the natural history of glomerulonephritis is unclear.

57) A) The description of the "one spot" as the starting point is the tip-off that pityriasis rosea is the diagnosis. This spot is called the "herald patch". While a herald patch can often be confused with tinea corporis, it would test negative on KOH preparation. They may also describe the rash distribution as a "Christmas tree" pattern.

58) D) All of the choices with the exception of toxic epidermal necrolysis (TEN) are associated with a bacterial exotoxin. TEN is a "hypersensitivity" reaction and involves full-thickness necrosis of the epidermal layer and deeper. This often results in pronounced erythema, which would also help distinguish this on the exam.

59) C) Given the description and distribution of the rash and the fact that the mother has a similar rash, the diagnosis is scabies. While antihistamines would be part of the treatment, it would not be the "most definitive" therapy for this condition. Always read the question, especially the last sentence, which contains the phrase indicating exactly what they are asking.

Endocrinology

60) C) Type 2 diabetes (insulin resistant) is being seen with greater frequency in the pediatric age group with an average age of onset of 12-1/2 vs. 7-1/2 for Type 1(insulin dependent). Type 2 diabetes is associated with obesity. Acanthosis nigricans (pigmentation in skin folds) is specifically associated with insulin resistance and is therefore more closely associated with type 2 diabetes. Metformin is an oral agent which decreases insulin resistance and is used to treat Type 2 diabetes. Both type 1 and type 2 are associated with hyperglycemia.

61) E) The most definitive way of distinguishing type 2 from type 1 diabetes melitis is to measure beta cell autoantibody levels. While diabetic ketoacidosis (DKA) is more common in type 1 disease it *can* present in type 2. A family history of type 2 disease would represent a risk factor for the same. However that does not mean a person with a strong family history of type 2 diseases, which is quite common could not develop type 1 anymore than if they came from a family with a strong history of owning little pink houses.

C-peptide correlates with insulin secretion could be low at initial presentation in both types and therefore cannot be used to *definitively* distinguish type 1 from type 2 disease.

Acanthosis nigricans is common in type 2, however obese individuals can also have insulin resistance **without having type 2 disease** therefore the presence of acanthosis nigricans cannot even confirm type 2 let alone be the way to definitively distinguish type 1 from type 2.

62) A) According to the American Diabetic Association, a diagnosis of diabetes can be established with:

· 2 hour post glucose challenge of 200 mg/dL or greater
> **OR**
· A random serum glucose of 200 mg/dL *plus symptoms*
> **OR**
· Fasting serum glucose of 126 mg/dL or greater **on 2 separate occasions**

This patient's fasting serum glucose of 110 does not meet the ADA criteria. However his 2 hour post glucose challenge does meet the criteria. A serum glucose of 230 is not life threatening and does not require the immediate implementation of oral hypoglycemic agents. Therefore the initial intervention would be nutrition and lifestyle changes with a one month followup. Waiting for symptoms to appear before followup would be inappropriate.

By the way some wrong answers are more wrong than others. Metformin would be the appropriate agent in children Glyburide as of this printing has not been approved for use in children.

63) E) Pubarche is the development of pubic hair, menarche is the onset of menses, thelarche is the beginning of breast development, and welders' arc is seen with professional welders who are hopefully past adolescence although not guaranteed.

While the timing of pubertal development can very from person to person, the sequence should not vary. Full development should not occur in one stage before the onset of the next stage. For example, a patient who experiences full breast development and no pubic hair deserves a workup. Therefore there should be partial thelarche not full thelarche before the onset of pubarche. Remember, menses occurs roughly two years after thelarche and pubarche a few *months* after thelarche.

64) D) If you chose F (16-1/2), then you did not memorize the definition of primary amenorrhea, which is no menses prior to age 16 if secondary sex characteristics are present and 14 years if secondary sex characteristics are absent.

65) C) Thyroxine levels do not go up during puberty. Insulin-like growth factor (IGF), testosterone, and estrogen levels are increased during puberty. Since global warming is all the rage one would have to assume water levels due to the polar ice cap melting is also rising. It would therefore also be occurring during pubertal development.

Remember to read the question carefully. In case the question is worded in such a way, thyroxine does serve as an agent that stimulates "skeletal maturation". Hypothyroidism, however, is one of the causes of short stature.

66) D) The growth spurt tends to occur later in boys than girls at SMR 4.

67) C) The growth spurt tends to occur earlier in girls than in boy at SMR 3.

68) A) Patient's who experience thyroid storm can also have liver disease and be jaundiced. However hepatomegaly is not seen in patient's who are hyperthyroid. Pretibial myxedema is common in adults not children who are hyperthyroid. While patients with Graves's disease can be exophthalmic, you may experience exophthalmia when you realize the absence of it does not rule out Graves's disease.

69) C) The onset of puberty in boys in marked by testicular enlargement (as well as elongation and thinning of the scrotum) and this is where the latest model orchidometer comes in handy (no pun intended). Remember for guys it's two buds (testes) getting bigger down low and for girls it's two (breast) buds getting bigger up top. Please insert you own Budweiser® Superbowl commercial here.

70) D) Thelarche is the endocrinologists' term for breast budding. This indeed is the first sign of pubertal development in females followed by pubarche (pubic hair) and then menarche 1 – 2 years later.

71) 1) (C)
      2) (B)
      3) (C)
      4) (D)
      5) (A)

Delayed bone age and family history apply to both hypothyroidism and constitutional growth delay. Parents of children with constitutional growth delay achieve normal height and the children can expect the same fate. In fact frequently the parent's have a similar history of delayed growth. Normal adult height applies only to constitutional growth delay. One would not expect normal adult height in patient's with precocious puberty especially if untreated since the growth plates will likely fuse prematurely.

72) It is important to take a long hard look at this curve since it can very likely appear on the exam.

1) (B) - Craniopharyngioma. After surgical correction at puberty, height can be expected to increase.

2) (C) - Hypothyroid. This curve is similar to craniopharyngiomas' curve; however, if they were to present both on the same graph, the hypothyroid would be the one presenting earlier. Growth resumes at the time of treatment.

3) (A) - Untreated congenital adrenal hyperplasia. These children grow rapidly but if they are not treated, their growth plates will fuse early. Look for a steady incline with a plateau effect early on. Note that the adult height will be shorter than expected based on mid parental height due to early fusion of the growth plates.

4) (D) - Constitutional delay. Here children remain on a short growth curve (unlike with hypothyroid, CAH and craniopharyngioma where they plateau out) but then experience the classic growth spurt.

5) (E) - Genetic short stature. In this case, children are on a short growth curve and stay there. They are "just plain short" and will be short adults.

73)
1) (C) - Blood volume. Notice that this curve more or less follows a standard growth curve. This applies to tissue that grows in proportion to normal growth. This is the same curve that would apply to **blood, liver, bone, pancreas** and other **organs that are <u>non-lymphoid.</u>**
2) (E) - **Spleen**. This is also the pattern for **tonsils** and **lymphoid tissue**. They reach their *peak around 12.*
3) (A) - **Thymus**. You see a *rapid decline just before puberty.*
4) (B) - **Testes**. This curve applies to any choice those results in *rapid growth around puberty.* Other choices they might present you will are uterus and ovary.\
5) (D) - **Skull. Brain, skull** and other **neural tissue** reach a *peak at around 4* when no additional growth is expected.

74a) C) This is a description of Turner syndrome, and all of the findings are likely associations except for 45, XXY, which would be Klinefelter's syndrome and not a variation of Turner's syndrome.

74b) D) *Growth hormone* and *oxandrolone* have been shown to improve final height in girls with Turner's syndrome and is approved by the FDA for this purpose. In fact, the use of combination GH and oxandrolone increases growth rate more than either agent alone. Although *estrogen* contributes to pubertal growth spurt, it also results in fusion of the epiphyseal plates and is *thus most effective when given later in puberty* (14-16). The patient in the vignette is 14 and therefore too young to receive estrogen.

75) C) Here is an example where hard-fast rules are not absolute. **One cannot assume that a question involving head trauma or resection involving the brain will always lead to SIADH as the answer.** It is always best to put the lab findings into words in the margins. The best explanation for the *hyperkalemia* would be secondary *adrenal insufficiency.*

76) A) The side effects of daily/long-term steroid use include growth retardation, adrenal suppression, cataracts, osteopenia, aseptic necrosis of the femoral head, glucose intolerance, and an increased risk of infection and cosmetic effects. **Memory loss is not a side effect of chronic steroid use.**

77) C) Given the fact that both parents "hover" around 5 feet and assuming that the parents had adequate nutrition in their youth and have reached close to their growth potential, this would be familial short stature or "just plain short". There is nothing in the history to suggest otherwise. If one of the parents had experienced a growth spurt, this would have to be noted in the question... Therefore constitutional growth delay would be a possibility, however in this question this is not noted and familial short stature is the correct answer.

78) C) Of all the choices listed the best estimate of this boy's adult height is the mean parental height **plus** 6.5 cm. For girls it is mean adult height minus 6.5 cm.

79) D) Of all the choices listed the best estimate of this girl's adult height is the mean parental height **minus** 6.5 cm. For boys it is mean adult height plus 6.5 cm.

80) D) This patient presents with *obesity, hirsutism,* and *irregular menses.* This is the classic triad of **polycystic ovary disease (Stein-Leventhal syndrome).**

Polycystic Ovaries develop when the ovaries are stimulated to produce excessive amounts of male hormones (androgens), particularly testosterone, either through the release of excessive luteinizing hormone (LH) by the anterior pituitary gland or through high levels of insulin in the blood (hyperinsulinemia) in women whose ovaries are sensitive to this stimulus.

Polycystic "obese" ovaries should help you remember to associate obesity with polycystic ovary syndrome.

ENT

81) D) The presentation is consistent with laryngomalacia, which improves with time and no intervention. Improvement occurs as the cartilage becomes stronger. Think of laryngomalacia when they describe stridor which improves on expiration.

82) E) However, if you had to pick just one answer it would be "pneumatic otoscopy"; that is the answer they are usually looking for. Since just "seeing red" is not reliable, you have to also see decreased movement of the tympanic membrane. Also, remember that decongestants are not a reliable way to prevent ear infections.

83) 1) (A)
2) (B)
3) (D)
4) (B)

Laryngomalacia would be described as inspiratory stridor, wet or otherwise. You can remember this as lar-IN-gomalacia.

Tracheomalacia would present as expiratory stridor. You can remember this as Trach-E-EX omalacia.

Tracheomalacia can occur after surgery to repair a tracheo-esophageal fistula.

84) D) *Epiglottitis* would be an example of "supraglottic" obstruction, which can present with drooling due to the diminished ability to swallow saliva. This is typically due to H. flu and is quite rare due to the success of the HiB vaccine. However like all other diseases eradicated through immunization, it can creep its way onto the boards where most patients are not immunized.

Epiglottitis can be a surgical emergency since the airway can rapidly close off. In general, the obstruction above the glottis improves **with expiration,** but can close down with inspiration since the negative pressure pulling down can collapse the airway. *Therefore, inspiratory stridor is more common* which improves with expiration should make you think of a supraglottic airway obstruction.

A retropharyngeal abscess would be a cause of supraglottic airway obstruction, which does present with the hot potato voice.

85)   Part 1: A)

Bacterial tracheitis is an acute _bacterial_ infection of the upper airway and does not involve the epiglottis. However, like epiglottitis and croup, bacterial tracheitis is capable of causing life-threatening airway obstruction. Typically, the child has a brassy cough, apparently as part of a viral laryngotracheobronchitis. _Bacterial tracheitis is often a secondary infection._ High fever and "toxicity" with respiratory distress may occur immediately or after a few days of apparent improvement.

Part 2: E)

Usual treatment for croup (e.g., mist, intravenous fluid, aerosolized racemic epinephrine) is ineffective. Intubation or tracheostomy is usually necessary. Initially, removal of secretions may provide some relief, but ultimately intubation is necessary. IV antibiotics are also necessary.

86)   B)   Inspiratory stridor in a newborn as described would be most consistent with laryngomalacia. A 3-month-old would not likely aspirate a foreign body.

87)   D)   It is important to realize that they will rarely refer to _laryngotracheitis_ as "viral croup". They will either describe it clinically or go by the infinitely more confusing name _laryngotracheitis_.

In addition to the typical "barking cough", some of the more important features to note are the typical age of onset of 12 months, the fact that the stridor is biphasic[4] and that the condition is often preceded by a URI, and the fact that there can even be a "lower respiratory wheezing" component to the respiratory distress. The latter is important to note so you are not fooled if they throw this into an otherwise typical description of viral croup.

An important similar diagnosis in the differential would be **_spasmodic croup_**. This is more of an allergic phenomenon, and there is **no seasonal variation**. As with spasmodic croup, there will be no fever and more of an abrupt onset with no preceding URI.

---

[4] Both an inspiratory and expiratory component.

88)   A)   All of the above can be responsible for *acute otitis media with effusion* with the exception of *Haemophilus* influenza *type B.* This is sort of a trick question[5] since it is the "nontypeable" species that of *Haemophilus* influenza that can cause acute otitis media with effusion. Again, it pays to read the question very carefully.

89)   B)   These lesions are indeed acquired during the birth process when the mother has vaginal condylomata. Surgery is not curative at all, and repeated laser excision is often needed when the lesions grow back after excision. Malignant degeneration is actually more likely *after* radiation treatment.

90)   A)   Inflammatory mediators play an important role in persistent middle ear effusion following otitis media infections. As a result, *increased* (rather than decreased) blood flow to the mucous membranes plays a role. Persistent infection is not usually a factor, and certainly myringotomy tubes would not be indicated.

991)   D)   The key words here are **firm, non-tender** and **several months' duration** (rather than acute onset). This virtually rules out the infectious etiologies listed, including paramyxovirus, which is the name mumps goes by when it wants to impress more exotic viruses at viral cocktail parties. Neoplastic disease is the correct choice.

92)   C)   Although it is rarely seen in clinical practice anymore, you must still be familiar with the clinical scenario of *Haemophilus* influenza epiglottitis. Let's face it; mumps and measles are also quite rare these days, yet they frequently appear on the boards. This is especially true in this case where they note that the child has not been immunized.

The combination of stridor, high fever, apprehension, and drooling makes epiglottitis very likely and therefore warrants the presence of an anesthesiologist familiar with intubating children under difficult situations (i.e., a swollen epiglottis). Patients with epiglottitis should be intubated in the OR by an anesthesiologist with ENT or pediatric surgery on standby.

---

[5] Not unlike that you might encounter on the exam.

93) A) Daily antibiotic prophylaxis has fallen into disfavor with growing concerns over development of pneumococcal resistance.

94) E) Either clindamycin or azithromycin would be appropriate antibiotics in a penicillin allergic 4 year old with a dental infection.

95) D) Vomiting and blurred vision would be a sign of suppurative intracranial complication and spread. This should be pretty straightforward and certainly fair game on the exam.

96) E) Evacuation of the hematoma would be top priority to prevent subsequent deformity of the pinna

97) C) Of all the bacteria listed Staph aureus is the most likely cause of chronic sinusitis. S pneumoniae and Moraxella catarrhalis can cause chronic sinusitis but they are not the most likely cause.

H. Flu nontypeable can also cause chronic sinusitis, but not H. Flu type b.

98) C) Another episode of otitis media in the past 3 months would make withholding of antibiotics inappropriate according to the SNAP protocol.

Additional criteria that make withholding of antibiotics inappropriate would include fever or symptoms of otitis media for more than 48 hours. Chronic conditions which might impede an immune response, toxic appearance, evidence of perforation or impending perforation.

Additional contraindications include poor parental understanding of the protocol and/or difficulty gaining access to a medical facility afterward.

99)   D) The right sided heart sounds coupled with recurrent sinopulmonary infection suggests a diagnosis of Kartagener's syndrome or cilia dysmotility syndrome and electron microscopic exam of the nasal mucosa would be most helpful in establishing the diagnosis.

ER

100)   C) Sodium bicarbonate cannot be administered via an ET tube. You can use the mnemonic LANE to help remember that lidocaine, atropine, Narcan and epinephrine can all be administered via an endotracheal tube.

101)   B) The clinical picture is the deciding factor in determining whether to discharge a child with bronchiolitis rather than the etiology. . However the use of racemic epinephrine could result in resumption of symptoms after initial improvement as a rebound effect. The latter is somewhat controversial however a period of observation of 6 hours and/ or an admission would be appropriate.

102)   B) An abuse pattern will more typically appear with different degrees of variation in shade and not be uniform in color (such as are Mongolian spots and the discoloration they are describing). The strawberry hemangiomas will typically become worse prior to involuting. No intervention is needed unless it is large enough and in an area that could potentially interfere with function, for example, near the eyelid where it would obstruct vision.

103) C) IV normal saline would be appropriate in treating acute methamphetamine toxicity.

However, beta-blockers alone should not be used because the unopposed alpha stimulation can be life threatening.

If reduction of blood pressure is the goal, an **alpha-blocker** such as **phentolamine** and a **vasodilator** such as **nifedipine** would be better choices.

Seizures can be controlled with benzodiazepines such as lorazepam.

Except for beta blockers all of the other choices can be indicated under certain conditions and be safely used to manage acute methamphetamine intoxications.

104) E) This child is exhibiting *Cushing's Triad*, which is seen in patients with increased intracranial pressure:

1. Hypertension
2. Bradycardia
3. Irregular respirations

A lumbar puncture would not only be unhelpful but contraindicated in the face of increased intracranial pressure. None of the other steps would address the main problem except for *hyperventilation*, which induces hypocarbia, resulting in cerebral vasoconstriction and decreased cerebral blood flow.

105) A) The clinical scenario is that of *opiate overdose*. Administering naloxone would initially be diagnostic (pupil dilating) and ultimately therapeutic as more is given once diagnosis is confirmed

Clearly glucose would be contraindicated in a patient who is already hyperglycemic.

106) C) Cardiac arrhythmias such as inverted T-waves and depressed ST segments would be the most "serious" consequences of glue sniffing. Management in the acute situation is directed toward monitoring for cardiac arrhythmias above all else.

107) E) Since this child is on chronic systemic steroids, adrenal suppression is very likely. Therefore, administering perioperative steroids IV would be indicated.

108) C) Administration of insulin and glucose would actually be an appropriate method to treat *hyperkalemia.* Cardiorespiratory monitoring would certainly be appropriate and necessary to monitor for any cardiac arrhythmias that might develop as a result of hypokalemia.

109) D) Although the typical presentation of pyelonephritis might be "flank pain" or CVA[6] tenderness, **pyelonephritis can also present as RUQ tenderness.** The other findings, including the positive lab culture with greater than 100,000 colonies of a typical pathogen, would suggest infection of the upper urinary tract and not just "cystitis".

There is nothing in this vignette to suggest renal stones.

110) D) Despite the relatively benign physical examination including a GCS of 14, the history of loss of consciousness coupled with the vomiting would warrant a CT scan. Overnight observation would be indicated as well, but the head CT would not be dependent on observed clinical status during the hospital stay, it would precede the admission.

111) A) This is a classic description of PCP (phencyclidine) ingestion. Hyperreflexia is associated with PCP ingestion.

With higher levels of PCP ingestion, patients can become comatose and hypotensive. *However, respiratory depression is rare and more consistent with opiate overdose.* .

---

[6] Costovertebral angle.

112) E) This is a *septal hematoma* and essentially a surgical emergency. If the hematoma is not evacuated and proper surgical intervention implemented, it will result in compromised blood supply to the cartilage and a *"saddle nose" deformity*. This is the typical deformity seen in old boxers and extras on the set of all of the "Rocky" movies.

113) C) Once again, rarely is something mentioned without a reason. The child has an unremarkable history and comes to the ER lethargic. **Noting that the mother is being treated for depression is important and suggestive of a toxic ingestion.**

Syrup of ipecac is no longer recommended for toxic ingestions, especially one who presents with CNS depression.

The most likely ingested medication is a tricyclic antidepressant which is a board favorite. Tricyclic ingestion can result in cardiac arrhythmias, making the EKG an appropriate step. Although not listed, alkalinization of the urine would also be appropriate.

Certainly, protecting the airway of a lethargic child could never be an incorrect choice. Once intubated, administration of charcoal via an NG tube could be indicated.

114) E) Answer E would be consistent with Caffey disease, which also goes by the name *infantile cortical hyperostosis*. A metaphyseal fracture,[7] also known as a "bucket handle" fracture, is virtually always secondary to abuse. While a child who is ice-skating may fall a lot, rib fractures are very unlikely to be "accidental" unless they were playing hockey against teenagers (the same would apply to a skull fracture). Although bruising of the shins is very common in 2-year-olds you would not expect to see evidence of "multiple fractures" unless there was a result of a non accidental injury.

115) A) Deferoxamine binds free iron in the serum and forms ferrioxamine, a water soluble, renally excreted compound which, if present, turns the urine a characteristic reddish-orange or "vin rose" color.

---

[7] Not to be confused with a metaphysical fracture, which is a fracture from reality!

116) C) The ultimate determination regarding whether sexual abuse has or has not occurred is a legal one determined by the court system. Of course the court system will consider evidence presented by the pediatrician and other specialists involved but ultimately it is a court decision.

117) E) Neglect is the most common form of child abuse.

118) C) Any child exhibiting vomiting and lethargy following a head injury requires prompt evaluation. Skull films have no place; it is either Head CT or no studies.

119) C) Domestic violence occurs in 13% of households in the general population. It occurs in 40-60% of households where physical abuse takes place. Fear of strangers including clinicians is a sign of domestic violence in the household.

In a household that experiences 50 or more episodes of domestic violence 30% of children will be abused by their mothers. There is a 150% increasein risk of child sexual abuse in households where domestic violence takes place.

120) C) Ketamine has the potential to *increase* not decrease secretions. Therefore, it is often used with atropine to counter this effect. It works primarily via sensory blockade and is often used for short painful procedures.

One of the problems with ketamine is it can produce a dreamlike state, with hallucinations *before* the sensory blockade takes effect. The last thing you want is a patient hallucinating in anticipation of a painful procedure. That is why midazolam is often used together with ketamine.

121) A) Midazolam's usefulness in conscious sedation is due to is, amnesic, anxiolytic, and sedative effects. It has *no analgesic effect*

I would say that anything which an anxiolytic, amnesic and sedating is quite enigmatic. The important point to remember I that midazolam has no analgesic benefits and if a procedure is painful another agent must be used as well.

122) C) The most common trigger for life threatening anaphylaxis in children is foods.

123) D) The most likely diagnosis would be intussusception. Intussusception presents between ages 3 months – 3 years, with intermittent episodes of vomiting with lethargy in between episodes in a child who is afebrile. In addition to the classic currant jelly stools, bilious vomiting could also be part of the presenting picture. On x-ray, specifically air or contrast enema can reveal the lead point as a "coiled spring" appearance.

If you see the words coiled spring in the description and intussusception as one of the answers, you can for all intents and purposes break out the cork screw to open the champagne en route to your taking another step toward passing the exam.

Fluids & Lytes

124) Part 1: B)

This patient is presenting with a hyponatremic **hypochloremic metabolic alkalosis**. It is a good idea to get in the habit of "*turning numbers into words*" and also *calculating the anion gap* when the components are presented to you. In this case the anion gap is 11 and not elevated. Congenital adrenal hyperplasia (CAH) will present with an elevated K, which is not the case here. In addition, CAH is associated with *low bicarb and elevated urine sodium* greater than 20mEq/L. The urine sodium concentration of 5 or less coupled with the BUN/CRE ratio of less than 20 all but rules out renal disease. Just plain cool headed thinking on the exam will allow you to rule out proximal tubular acidosis based on the lab values presented in the history. The patient is *alkalotic* not *acidotic*.

Part 2: D

Hyponatremic hypochloremic metabolic alkalosis is associated with cystic fibrosis and any infant presenting with it should have a **sweat chloride** done to rule it out.

125) 1) (F)
2) (E)
3) (D)
4) (C)
5) (B)
6) (A)

Explanation: This is another board classic that is asked every year so know it well. Here is the logic tree to make it easy.

Lab error

If you note low **sodium** but a **normal chloride**, this is lab error.

True hyponatremic dehydration includes a low serum chloride in addition to low serum sodium. This is consistent with choice C.

Pseudohyponatremia The key findings are low serum sodium with a high glucose (or albumen, mannitol or anything that takes up "serum space" instead of water).

SIADH and diabetes insipidus (DI) are easy to confuse in the line of fire. Remember that **SIADH** results in *fluid retention* and therefore low serum sodium with *inappropriately concentrated urine.*

DI is the opposite. This can be thought of as "inappropriate urine production" resulting in high serum sodium and very dilute urine. Keeping these facts straight should make the fluid grid a point grab on the exam.

126) E) **Furosemide** inhibits the reabsorption of sodium and chloride in the proximal part of the loop of Henle. This promotes excretion of sodium, chloride, water, and potassium.[8] Therefore, the answer would be **hypochloremia** and **hypokalemia,** regardless of whether the patient was taking digoxin as well.

---

[8] No relation to Don Henley, formerly of the Eagles.

127) E) A systematic approach to this type of question makes it an easy one. Clearly the pH is normal, so there is some sort of compensation, eliminating lab error as an option. Respiratory acidosis with respiratory compensation makes as much sense as a 6 foot 11 inch jockey.

With bicarb of 18 you are looking at *metabolic acidosis that has been compensated by a respiratory effort* (tachypnea) to blow off CO_2, thus explaining the PCO_2 of 30.

128) C) This patient is presenting with signs of *clinical shock*. A 0.9% Normal Saline bolus 20 cc/kg would be the most prudent "next" step. Normal Saline would be an isotonic solution and most appropriate to treat the hypovolemia this patient is experiencing.

Administer 0.9% Normal Saline, isotonic solution, 20 cc/kg over 20 minutes would be another appropriate choice.

129) A) This concentration for oral rehydration therapy is chosen because it allows for maximal absorption of sodium through or via the sodium-glucose cotransporter. This is an important point that is frequently tested on the Boards.

130) C) Whenever you are presented with a head injury, tumor, or neurosurgical case, coupled with a fluid and electrolyte imbalance, always consider **SIADH** first.

This is certainly the correct diagnosis here. SIADH is the "inappropriate" secretion of ADH (anti-diuretic hormone). Therefore, urination is inappropriately diminished and fluid is retained. This explains the low sodium[9] and **need for fluid restriction**.

131) C) By convention potassium is ignored in the calculation of plasma osmolality since its contribution is negligible.

---

[9] Remember to write the word hyponatremia in the margin.

132) E)   In congestive heart failure, the primary abnormality is sodium retention. Patients present with increased body weight due to retained water.

Water is retained to maintain osmolality within normal range. Edema is commonly seen depending on the degree of sodium retention.

Despite this *Normal serum sodium is maintained.*

133) C)   This patient has a normal gap Sodium – (Chloride+ Bicarb) which in this case would be 15 ruling out diabetic ketoacidosis and alcoholic acidosis which would not be expected in a child this age. Congenital adrenal hyperplasia would present with hyperkalemia. There is also no evidence of pulmonary hypertension.

The combined lab findings of metabolic acidosis and failure to thrive make renal tubular acidosis the most likely diagnosis.

134) B)   Laxative abuse, diuretic therapy, Gitelman syndrome and Bartter syndrome are all associated with metabolic alkalosis

Organophosphate poisoning is associated with *respiratory acidosis.*

135) **D)**   Arteriole constriction, reduced coronary blood flow hypokalemia and hypoventilation are all consequences of severe alkalemia.

However hypocapnia would not be a consequence of severe alkalemia. In fact hypoventilation in response to alkalemia would result in hypercapnia.

136) C)   The clinical presentation and lab findings are consistent with a diagnosis of pyloric stenosis and the most appropriate study would be an abdominal ultrasound.

137) A) With **heat stress** one would see decreased exercise performance but little else

With **heat exhaustion** one would see confusion, nausea, vomiting and a core temperature between 100.4 F and 104.

With **heat stroke** one would see a core temperature greater than 104 F.

Genetics

138) A) Gardner's syndrome results in supernumerary teeth (i.e., extra teeth). All of the other choices are associated with a delayed eruption of teeth. E is not exactly correct; since most hockey players are missing teeth but not secondary to delayed eruption of teeth.

139) B) Mental Retardation. Here is an example where good test taking skills might come in handy. Choices C and E are linked and can be eliminated narrowing it down to 3 choices. See the Treacher Collins (Teacher Calling) section of the Genetics chapter in our main text.

140) B) Aicardi syndrome is one of the few disorders that are inherited in an X-linked *dominant* fashion.

Therefore it is an x-linked disease which *can* appear in females because it is a dominant trait on the X chromosome. Another feature of Aicardi syndrome is an absent corpus callosum.

141) C) Trisomy 18 is associated with clenched fist, rocket bottom feet, prominent occiput and horseshoe kidney. It is also associated with overlapping fingers which has a "clenched fist" appearance. Trisomy 18 is not aassociated with bicornate uterus.

142) C) This is an autosomal dominant trait, and therefore all children have a 50% chance of having the disorder, regardless of gender. Don't be tricked by a decoy choice that splits the pattern based on gender. Remember if Mom has the disorder she cannot be a carrier, and the disorder is not X-linked recessive. Noting which parent has the disorder will give you such clues.

143) C) Scalp defects, congenital heart defects, microphthalmia, and holoprosencephaly are all seen in Patau syndrome (Trisomy 13). Rocker bottom feet is seen with Edwards's syndrome (trisomy 18). Holoprosencephaly by the way is a single-lobed brain structure with severe skull and facial defects

144) D) 2/3. Here you would have to know that CF is an autosomal recessive disease. Since this is an *autosomal* recessive trait, the gender is irrelevant. Mentioning that this is a sister is therefore irrelevant. Go ahead and toss that red herring aside. The sister is unaffected, so if you run your Punnett square, you will get 3 possibilities for her: 1 possibility is disease free, no carrier and the other 2 possibilities are disease free, carrier, leaving you the answer 2/3 = 66%.

145) A) Wide gap between first and second toe, duodenal atresia, redundant skin on the posterior neck and palmar simian crease are consistent with Down syndrome, cleft lip and palate are not.

146) E) BH_4 is a cofactor for the enzyme *phenylalanine hydroxylase* which is required for tetrahydrobiopterin to break down phenylalanine into tyrosine. Therefore tetrahydrobiopterin deficiency can be present with a positive PKU test and clinical deterioration can present even when normal phenylalanine levels are maintained. It is also important to remember that tetrahydrobiopterin is the same as BH4 and they are interchangeable.. All documented cases of PKU should be followed up with testing for BH4 deficiency. By the way, A is correct but not the best answer.

147) A) Since this hemophilia A is an X-linked recessive disorder and the father is unaffected, his X chromosomes are also unaffected. Therefore, none of his offspring will be affected and the correct answer is 0%.

125% is the effort put forth by many professional ballplayers when they state "Everyone on this ball club is giving a 125% effort to win.

148) E) This is an example of a disorder inherited through DNA found in the mitochondria (in the cytoplasm as in non–nuclear DNA). This is inherited strictly in a **matrilineal inheritance** pattern. This is easy to remember if they ask any questions on the inheritance of disorders having to do with abnormalities in mitochondrial DNA. **M**atrilineal and **m**itochondrial both begin with **M**.

149) C) This is Prader-Willi syndrome, which may have confused you into choosing E, which is Slick Willy syndrome. Deletion on chromosome 15 leads to Prader-Willi syndrome when inherited from the father. Prader Willi can also be the result of maternal disomy where both number 15 chromosomes come from the mother

When the deletion occurs on the mother's number 15 chromosome the patient has Angelman syndrome. Angelman syndrome can also be a result of paternal disomy where both number 15 chromosomes come from the father.

Remember **P**rader is due to **p**aternal deletion and Angel**ma**n is due to **ma**ternal deletion.

150) C) Tuberous sclerosis is inherited in an autosomal dominant pattern.

151)   1)   (B)
            2)   (A)
            3)   (C)
            4)   (A)
            5)   (C)

Noonan was and is sometimes referred to as "male Turner's". This is a misnomer. Turner's affects genetic females only but Noonan can occur in both males and females. They share *some* phenotypical similarities, but they are quite different. Turner's is X/O (with a variety of mosaic variations) and Noonan syndrome has no identifiable genetic pattern.

152)   C)   1 in 150. is the correct answer.

Here you need to know that the carrier rate for CF in the general population is 1/25 (basically the only one you will need to memorize) and that CF is autosomal recessive. The sibling has a 2/3 chance of being a carrier. You can work this through logically using the Punnett Square or you can just memorize it. When 2 carriers get together there is a 1/4 chance of having a child with CF.

Putting it all together you get 1 in 150 as the correct answer to this question.
$(1/25) \times (2/3) \times (1/4) = 1/1150$

GI

153)   D)   Small bowel biopsy is the definitive test for gluten sensitive enteropathy. If the question asked for the most appropriate initial step than a *Transglutaminase Antibody (tTG)* measure would be more appropriate.

Another example where reading the question is critical to answering it correctly.

154) B) One of the hallmarks of chronic non-specific diarrhea is *normal growth.* In fact, if this is described in the question, circle it; there are few forms of chronic diarrhea in the differential that *don't* affect growth and this is one of them. None of the other descriptions are associated with chronic non-specific diarrhea including flatulence of any kind, let alone to the point of having guests leaving on schedule.

155) A) A stool pH less than 5 and positive reducing substances suggest carbohydrate malabsorption, which is not the cause of toddler's diarrhea.

Watery diarrhea with occult blood, absence of diarrhea overnight with an increase incidence in the morning is all consistent with a diagnosis of chronic non specific diarrhea.

Note that grossly "bloody stools" are inconsistent with the diagnosis; "occult blood" would be consistent. Occult blood often occurs with perianal irritation and/or excoriation from the chronic diarrhea.

156) 1) (C)
2) (F)
3) (D)
4) (E)

Fecal impaction will frequently be presented as left lower quadrant fullness.

However partial small bowel obstruction would present as vomiting, weight loss and anorexia.

Crohn's disease would be presented as pressure tenderness on the right lower quadrant along with systemic findings such as fever and joint aches.

Mesenteric venous obstruction could be seen in a teenager using oral contraceptives.

157) 1) (A)
         2) (C)
         3) (B)

Not only is surgery not curative with Crohn's but it can also accelerate the reoccurrence process.

Both Crohn's disease and ulcerative colitis are associated with ankylosing spondylitis. Surgery is only curative for ulcerative colitis not Crohn's disease.

158) E) Whenever you see signs of **pancreatic insufficiency in an infant coupled with anemia,** think of Shwachman-Diamond syndrome. This is an autosomal *recessive* disorder which presents with poor growth and greasy, foul smelling stools that are characteristic of malabsorption. The pancreatic insufficiency is often transient, and can resolve by age 4.

Cyclical neutropenia is another associated finding. **Skeletal abnormalities** such as metaphyseal dysostosis[10] are also common in Shwachman-Diamond syndrome.

This should not be confused with Diamond-Blackfan syndrome,[11] which also presents with anemia in infancy, but without signs of malabsorption. **The normal sweat chloride tests rules out cystic fibrosis,** another possible cause of malabsorption in infants.

159) E) Diagnostic studies such as pH probe studies would be limited to complicated cases, e.g., blood-tinged emesis or apnea.

160) B) While projectile vomiting can occur with GE reflux, it is not *the most common symptom.* Likewise, while both apnea and aspiration pneumonia can occur with GE reflux, they also are not *the most common symptoms*, and poor weight gain is very unlikely with uncomplicated GE reflux.

The most common symptom of gastroesophageal reflux in infants is recurrent regurgitation.

---

[10] Whatever that is but very different than metaphysical dysostosis
[11] Congenital hypoplastic anemia.

161) D) Tocopherol is vitamin E, which is responsible for cell membrane stabilization. Deficiency of vitamin E often results in red cell hemolysis, particularly in premature infants. Vitamin E deficiency can also impair nerve cell integrity and can result in neurological symptoms as well.

162) E) Anorexia, slowed growth, drying and cracking of the skin, hepatosplenomegaly, and increased intracranial pressure can all be the result of excess intake of *retinol,* or vitamin A.

It can also result in carotenemia. Consider diet as the cause of yellow colors in a child that is non-icteric.[12] In these questions they will often describe excess intake of carrots, squash, and other foods rich in beta-carotene. In other words, don't choose until you've seen the "yellow described in the eyes".

163) E) Cyanocobalamin is the formal name for vitamin B12. The failure to absorb vitamin B12 can result in or be the result of **any condition that interferes with the absorption of B12.**

This includes
· Juvenile pernicious anemia
· Celiac disease
· Methylmalonic aciduria.

B12 deficiency is also associated with homocystinuria. In addition, metabolism of nervous tissue can be impaired, resulting in neurological abnormalities; macrocytic anemia can result as well.

164) 1) (C)
2) (A)
3) (D)
4) (B)

Explanation: **GE reflux** is often a normal finding in newborns; therefore, reassurance is often all that is needed. **Rumination** is associated with emotional deprivation and rarely occurs during the night. **Duodenal atresia** is associated with diminished fetal ingestion of amnionic fluid, resulting in poly-hydramnios. It is important to remember that **necrotizing enterocolitis** can occur in full-term infants, and it should be considered when presented with a full-term infant with classic signs of necrotizing enterocolitis.

---

[12] This would be evident by yellow-colored skin without yellow sclera.

165) 1) (A)
2) (D)
3) (E)
4) (C)
5) (B)

Explanation: Vomiting secondary to a neurological cause can be the result of an *intracranial hemorrhage*, resulting in a rapid drop of the hematocrit.

Gastroesophageal reflux can accompany neurological signs such as posturing. *Sandifer syndrome*, which is not included in the question but could appear on the exam, can present with both vomiting and torticollis.

Rumination is primarily a behavioral disorder; therefore, behavioral interventions can often be the treatment of choice.

It is important to distinguish gastrointestinal cow milk allergy from allergic gastroenteropathy. **Allergic gastroenteropathy** is also termed *eosinophilic gastroenteritis*. Eosinophilic gastroenteritis can present with atopy in addition to weight loss, hypoalbuminemia, and diarrhea.

Cow milk allergy can present with chronic respiratory problems, rhinitis, colic, and even occult blood loss...

This can occur in a breast feeding child if the mother is ingesting mild protein products.

166) A) Wilson disease is inherited in an autosomal recessive pattern. It can present with a mixed conjugated and unconjugated hyperbilirubinemia and rarely presents before age 3.

In addition to D-penicillamine trientine is also a copper chelator. Zinc acetate prevents absorption of copper from the GI tract.

167) D) Feeding refusal, poor weight gain, apnea and upper airway symptoms are all complications of GERD in infants.

Anemia could be a symptom of GERD in older children possibly in association with hematemesis but not in infants.

168) D) Delayed gastric emptying is an important factor in the vomiting seen during acute rotavirus infection.

All of the other statements are true. Fomites formation plays a major role in transmission of disease. The rotavirus is quite a sturdy little virus, remaining active awaiting its next victim on porous surfaces especially toilet handles and sinks. That it is why it is worth using a paper towel when opening the door to leave a public bathroom

Rotavirus infection is seen during the colder winter months and *has* been isolated from the respiratory tract. Often respiratory symptoms accompany the GI symptoms. Adults are more likely to be asymptomatic when infected with the virus.

169) A) Abdominal migraines can present as episodic periumbilical or epigastric pain. The pain is acute and can last an hour or more and there is often a positive family history.

It is occurs more frequently in *females.*

GU

170) E) The child in the vignette is experiencing primary enuresis that occurs independent of activity or time of day, suggesting an anatomic etiology. There is nothing in the history to suggest diabetes insipidus and nothing on history or physical to suggest a neurogenic bladder. Likewise, there is nothing in the history to suggest giggling incontinence or UTI.

The MOST likely explanation would be an ectopic uretal orifice resulting in dribbling.

171) C) The risk of malignancy in the undescended testis is 4 to 10 times higher than that in the general population. Surgical correction (orchiopexy) does not change the risk of developing cancer of the testis. Boys with a retractile testis are not at increased risk for infertility or malignancy.

Retractile testicles which can be brought down the scrotum need no additional intervention. It certainly cannot go back up resulting in cryptorchidism. It is a one way elevator ride, once testicle hit the ground floor they do not go back up.

Self- examination of the testes is important given the increased risk for malignancy when cryptorchidism is corrected with orchiopexy.

172) E) The mean penile length during the first 5 months of age in a term baby is 3.9cm and 4.1 cm is well within that range. Therefore delicate reassurance of the father is in order.

173) D) Even though in the real word documentation of bilateral descended testicle may not be correct, on the boards any statement not placed in quotes can be considered to be absolute.

You have a testicle which cannot be palpated in a child with previously documented bilateral descended testicles. Since this is a down elevator only the only logical next step would be to reposition and re-examine the patient.

174) D) The question did not mention when her last menstrual period was or if she was sexually active.

Certainly any fertile female presenting with a 2-week history of nausea and vomiting before anything else should have pregnancy ruled out first and foremost .

175) D) True bacterial epididymitis is rare in children. Nausea and vomiting are rarely seen in epididymitis which occurs over days rather than hours.

The blue dot sign distinguishes torsion of the testicular appendage from testicular torsion and not the other way around. Torsion of the testicular appendage is treated conservatively with NSAID, warm compresses, and reduced physical activity.

Inguinal hernia can indeed present with acute scrotal pain and/or swelling.

Heme One

176) C) Hyperphosphatemia, hyperkalemia, and hyperuricemia are all seen in tumor lysis syndrome. Alkalinization is part of the treatment.

However hypernatremia is not associated with tumor lysis syndrome.

177) B) Reed-Sternberg cells, non tender cervical nodes, elevated white blood cell count, and low lymphocyte count are associated with Hodgkin's lymphoma.

A rapidly growing non-tender abdominal mass is more typical of non-Hodgkin's lymphoma.

178) B) Neutropenia is an absolute neutrophil count less than 1500. Just memorize it, that's the way it is

179) E) G6PD deficiency is an X-linked recessive disorder. The best explanation would be for the mother and father to have both passed on an X gene for G6PD deficiency to their daughter.

180) B) The average period between neutropenic episodes is 3 weeks with each episode lasting several days.

181) 1) (A) Chediak-Hitachi syndrome.
2) (B) Chronic granulomatous disease.
3) (D) Leukocyte adhesion deficiency.
4) (C) Cyclic neutropenia.
5) (E) Shwachman-Diamond syndrome

Chediak-Hitachi syndrome is associated with lysosomal granules.

Chronic granulomatous disease is associated with chronic Staph in fections.

Leuckocyt adhesion deficiency is associated with delayed sepration of the umbilical stump.

Cyclic neutropenia is associated with Clostridium perfingens infection.

Shwachman-Diamone syndrome is associated with pancreatic insufficiency.

182) 1) (A)
2) (B)
3) (A)
4) (D)

Anemia of chronic illness presents with a low iron binding capacity and high serum ferritin.

Iron deficiency presents with a high iron binding capacity and a low serum ferritin.

Neither one presents with a low MCV and a low RDW. Iron deficiency is a microcytic anemia and presents with a low MCV, however it has a high RDW. Anemia of chronic illness is typically a normocytic anemia.

In **iron deficiency anemia,** the **TIBC** is high. Think of iron binding capacity as trucks to transport iron where it is needed. When there isn't a lot of iron around, as is the case with iron deficiency anemia, there are plenty of truck waiting around and the iron binding capacity is high. Serum iron stores or serum ferritin is low in iron deficiency anemia.

However, with **anemia of chronic illness,** there isn't a lot of iron around and the trucks also don't have any gas, so they remain in the garage, so the iron binding capacity is low. Since the reserves were there before the illness, **serum ferritin** is high in anemia of chronic illness.

183) 1) (C)
2) (D)
3) (D)

Hemophilia A and B are both X-linked recessive disorders. Mucosal bleeds are common in von Willebrand's disease and not Hemophilia A or B.

184) 1) (A)
2) (B)
3) (D)
4) (D)

Ewing sarcoma is uncommon in African Americans.

Osteogenic sarcoma will often present with a history of trauma to the involved bone, followed by persistent pain.

The description of "pain worse at night relieved by ibuprofen" is typical of osteoma osteoid, a benign tumor.

In past years this was described as pain relieved by aspirin. However it seems that finally this has been updated to reflect that the use of aspirin in children has been phased out with 1970's rotary phones.

The last description is of Homer Simpson.

185)   1)   (A)
            2)   (B)
            3)   (C)
            4)   (B)
            5)   (A)
            6)   (A)

Diamond Blackfan syndrome (DBS) is a macrocytic anemia is due to an arrest in the maturation of red cells which occurs primarily in the newborn period. DBS is often treated with steroids and does *not* spontaneously resolve.

Transient erythroblastopenia of childhood (TEC) is a normocytic anemia due to the suppression of erythroid production. It is a condition which almost always resolves spontaneously. TEC is seen primarily in toddlers

Both TEC and DBS involve the red cell line primarily.

186)   E)   With a question like this, which is heavy in the lab data and seemingly irrelevant bits of information, it is important to put the findings into words in the margins. With that information you can systematically narrow down the diagnostic choices.

You should note a **"recent URI"**, normocytic anemia, WBC, platelets, and retic count all within normal limits. No liver or spleen palpated on the physical exam.

With a normal liver, spleen, and retic count, you have *already ruled out a hemolytic anemia-like G6PD deficiency, as well as sickle cell disease.*

The labs are consistent with a **normocytic anemia.** Which *rules out iron deficiency anemia* and thalassemia.

The normal WBC and platelets rule out aplastic anemia.

This narrows you down to two choices: Diamond-Blackfan anemia and transient erythroblastopenia. *Diamond-Blackfan is primarily seen in infants* younger than 6 months. Given the recent URI, presumed to be of viral origin, you are left with transient erythroblastopenia.

187) D) Children with neuroblastoma can sometimes, especially on the boards, present with **opsoclonus-myoclonus,** which are myoclonic jerking and random movements of the eyes described in this question.

These findings combined with the abdominal mass makes neuroblastoma the most likely diagnosis.

188) C) With anemia secondary to chronic illness, **marrow iron stores are actually *increased*.**

While the stores are increased, the iron is not released and is therefore unavailable for hemoglobin synthesis. In *anemia of chronic illness*, the **serum ferritin levels are elevated** and the serum iron binding capacity is reduced. It can present as a microcytic anemia, and therefore the MCV is low.

189) D) Since this is a *female* patient you should note in the margins that an X-linked recessive disorder is unlikely.

Factor VIII deficiency is an X-linked trait therefore Factor VIII deficiency is already ruled out. The history is, suggestive of *von Willebrand's disease* since this disorder is not sex linked and *can* affect females. Therefore a workup for *von Willebrand's disease* would be appropriate.

The workup would include bleeding time, prothrombin time, partial thromboplastin time (PTT), and von Willebrand's factor levels.

190) E) Any question involving "severe" seborrheic dermatitis coupled with otorrhea would suggest Langerhans' histiocytosis. The additional findings of polydipsia and polyuria suggest diabetes insipidus, another feature of Langerhans' cell histiocytosis.

191) D) Of all the disorders listed, xeroderma pigmentosum has the highest potential for malignant transformation. It is an autosomal recessive disorder, and the underlying defect is in the repair of DNA damaged by ultraviolet light. Exposure to ultraviolet light must be avoided, and vigilance for any skin changes is warranted.

192) C) If one parent had retinoblastoma, then there is a 50% chance that the child will have it. Fifteen percent of the cases are unilateral and hereditary, and 25% of the cases are bilateral and hereditary. Therefore, 40% of the cases are hereditary making it the neoplasm with the strongest familial tendency of the ones listed in the question.

193) D) Abdominal pain, nausea, and vomiting, coupled with the jaundice in a child with sickle cell disease should make you think about gallbladder disease.

Intermittent pain for 5 months, would suggest gallstones as the etiology of the pain.

Therefore, an abdominal ultrasound would be the study of choice.

Gallstone formation with associated abdominal pain is common in children with sickle cell disease.

194) B) Although severe, especially chronic fatigue, extramedullary hematopoiesis and growth retardation could be indications for transfusion in patients with hereditary spherocytosis, the *most common indication* would be *aplastic crisis* induced by Parvovirus B-19.

195) D) Hereditary spherocytosis is inherited *primarily* in an autosomal dominant pattern. It is not inherited exclusively in this pattern. In up to 25% of cases it appears as a spontaneous mutation in people with no prior family history.

Make sure you read the question very carefully, if they phrased it as "It is *exclusively* an autosomal dominant pattern" this would not be correct.

By the way, you can remember that it is autosomal dominant by changing SpherOcytosis to SpherDOcytosis, to remember it is autosomal Dominant. [13]

---

[13] X- Linked dominant disorders are so rare that it will be difficult to confuse which form of dominant inheritance this represents.

196) C) Splenectomy is generally *not* recommended in patients *younger than* 5. Partial splenectomy has been found to help reduce hemolysis while providing some protection against infection. The risk for infection is *highest during the first few months after splenectomy.*

A splenectomy would be indicated in a patient with splenomegaly if they wanted to participate in sports.

197) D) Cyclophosphamide increases the risk for developing bladder cancer as a secondary malignancy. It also causes hemorrhagic cystitis the reason why copious IV fluids are given during treatment.

198) D) Erythrocyte folic acid concentration is a better measurement of folic acid level "sufficiency" than folic acid levels.

One must first rule out B12 deficiency since if B12 deficiency is present treatment with folic acid will delay the diagnosis and perhaps lead to neurological sequelae.

199) D) It is easy to be diverted into believing this is thrombocytopenia absent radius syndrome (TA) however in TAR they would have to describe the absence of radius with the presence of a thumb. In addition since Fanconi anemia can present with hyperpigmented patches, short stature and skeletal abnormalities. This should be an easy diagnosis to make.

200) E) The chronicity of the pain coupled with the description of the multiple cysts should raise suspicions of ovarian cancer making serum markets to rule out ovarian cancer the correct answer.

ID

201) D) This is consistent with the Jarisch-Herxheimer reaction, in the past more commonly associated with the treatment of syphilis but also seen in the treatment of Lyme disease. It is due to lysis of the organism and the release of endotoxin.

202) E) The clinical scenario described is classic for Rocky Mountain spotted fever caused by *Rickettsia rickettsii.* **Note that the child did not visit the Rocky Mountains.** *That will never be included in the question.* They will mention the southeastern United States or east coast locations like Long Island. There are no lab tests available that would be helpful in the acute phase and immediate treatment is crucial; therefore, choice A would be inappropriate (serological tests wouldn't be available for 1-2 weeks). Broad-spectrum antibiotics are ineffective against *Rickettsia rickettsii* so IM ceftriaxone is inappropriate as well, eliminating choice B. Choice C may be correct but they are looking for the "best" answer. That leaves choice D or E. Both are appropriate treatment for Rocky Mountain spotted fever. Doxycycline would be the correct answer regardless of age. This is because staining of teeth is dose related and of secondary consideration regarding risk benefit ratio. Doxycycline is effective against ehrlichiosis and chloramphenicol may not be.

203) C) When orchitis presents as a complication of mumps it is typically unilateral. All of the other choices are consistent with a diagnosis of mumps.

204) B) Unlike in adults, TB is often "silent" in children, which makes screening in high-risk groups particularly important. This is the case even when presented with other symptoms consistent with TB such as cervical adenitis.

205) A) Of all the drugs listed only ethambutol is associated with optic neuritis.

206) D) The symptoms described are consistent with **cat scratch disease**. **Bartonella henselae** is the causative agent. Their noting her playing in the friend's backyard is important since that is where she most likely contracted the disease.

After an incubation period of 7–12 days,[14] one or more 3–5 mm red papules develop at the site of cutaneous inoculation, often reflecting a linear cat scratch. **Chronic regional lymphadenitis is the hallmark**, affecting the first or second set of nodes draining the entry site. Other nonspecific symptoms include malaise, anorexia, fatigue, and headache.

Unilateral conjunctivitis is a common "atypical"[15] finding. Presumably, direct eye inoculation occurs when hands touch the eye after touching a cat.

207) 1) (C)
2) (C)
3) (A)
4) (D)
5) (C)

Remember, both strep pharyngitis and infectious mononucleosis can present with exudative pharyngitis, high fever with enlarged tonsils, and group a beta hemolytic strep positive culture. A positive culture can also be seen with chronic carriers. Atypical lymphs, not atypical neutrophils, are found with mono; that is why it is important to read the question, or else you risk making a careless error because you read the question too quickly.

208) B) The clinical vignette is that of *typhoid fever*. While much of what is described is non-specific, the "rose spots" are often described in patients with typhoid fever.

Serological tests for *Salmonella* agglutinins (febrile agglutinins = the Widal test) are not recommended because of frequent false-negative and -positive results. Isolation of the *Salmonella* organism from the foci of infection is the most reliable test to make the diagnosis. Therefore, blood culture is the "first test" to order.

---

[14] Range 3–30 days.

[15] Yes, it is described as a "common" atypical finding, and many would argue that this is an oxymoron or a contradiction in terms. But such is life in the "semantic" world of medicine.

209) E) Antibiotics are not indicated with "uncomplicated" *Salmonella*. That would apply in this case since the patient is now afebrile and the blood cultures were negative, indicating "non-invasive" disease. Antibiotics would not shorten the duration of the disease and in fact might induce the carrier state.

Antibiotics *are* recommended only in children at risk for invasive disease. This would include infants younger than 3 months of age. The child in the vignette is 9 months old. If indicated, all of the antibiotics listed except erythromycin would be appropriate.

210) D) Because of the rarity of subsequent cases and the low risk of invasive group A *Strep* infections, routine prophylaxis is not recommended for school contacts. However, if the child should become symptomatic then a throat culture would certainly be appropriate.

211) C) Here it is important to read the question carefully. The key word is "routinely". While steroids are sometimes used in infectious mono, they are only used with markedly enlarged tonsils and possible respiratory compromise. Corticosteroids can also be used for acute urticaria but not routinely. Corticosteroids are not used to treat Kawasaki disease or toxic shock syndrome.

Corticosteroids are used routinely to manage tuberculosis meningitis to reduce the mortality and long-term neurological sequelae secondary to inflammation and increased intracranial pressure.

212) A) The mechanism of action of the botulism toxin is to block the release of acetylcholine from the *presynaptic* neuron.

Gentamicin and other aminoglycosides have been known to enhance "neuromuscular blockade." Therefore, gentamicin would be contraindicated in an infant admitted for botulism poisoning. In addition antibiotics in general are not used to treat infantile botulism. Treatment is largely supportive. **Constipation is a very early sign** and often precedes all other signs; *it is not a late finding.*

Last but not least, the active ingredient in Botox® injections is indeed botulism toxin; thus the name "Botox". It is used by plastic surgeons to reduce facial wrinkling. Apparently it does so by paralyzing muscle tissue. So much for function over vanity.

213) D) The only child who would legitimately be excused from school would be the child with *Strep* throat who is still febrile.

In general, a child with *Strep* throat should be kept from attending school until he is afebrile for 24 hours and/or has been treated with appropriate antibiotics for 24 hours.

Asymptomatic Salmonella gastroenteritis does not require exclusion from school.

Infectious mononucleosis does not preclude a child from attending class; the risk for spreading it to classmates is very low.

214) E) Three of the drugs listed are recommended to treat tularemia. However ciprofloxacin has been used effectively in a limited number of cases even though its use has not been approved in children younger than 18.

Doxycycline would not be appropriate in a child younger than 8 due to the risk for dental staining especially in a child when there are alternative medications that are approved in children younger than 8.

Gentamicin would be an appropriate first line medication in this child.

215) B) Ototoxicity correlates most with high peak levels. Peak levels are best obtained once a steady state is obtained. This occurs after the third dose, and the peak levels are determined 30 minutes after the dose is given.

216) D) Paronychia is the inflammation of the nail bed, or periungual skin.

An *acute* paronychia is often the result of chronic overzealous nail biting. This would be characterized by redness, swelling, and sometimes purulent discharge.

However, *chronic* paronychia noted in this question would present as edema and inflammation but not necessarily purulent discharge. Chronic paronychia is most likely due to *Candida albicans* or mouth flora and is often a result of thumb sucking. It is the chronic exposure to moisture that causes the problem.

217) C) Sometimes what you think is an obvious answer isn't. It would be conceivable that croup would require droplet precautions if pertussis does. In fact croup requires *contact precautions* primarily because of respiratory secretions. This is as good a time as any to emphasize that whenever they ask what is the best way to prevent the spread of *any* infection, the most likely answer will be hand washing.

218) B) Rifampin prophylaxis is recommended for household contacts, especially young children and childcare and nursery contacts during the previous 7 days. Of course, anyone who came into direct contact with body secretions[16] would also be treated with rifampin prophylaxis.

While it won't factor into the exam, you should warn folks on rifampin of the strange electric-orange color their urine will take on. It can stain contact lenses and more importantly can interfere with the efficacy of oral contraceptive pills, anti- seizure meds, and some anticoagulants.

219) A) Don't be so quick to jump on the group A beta-hemolytic *Strep* bandwagon while ignoring the possibility of a "virus", Adenovirus to be exact. Adenovirus is the most likely cause of the above set of symptoms. This is especially so during the summer, and on the exam.

220) D) This is a classic presentation of *Staph* pneumonia. It initially manifests as upper respiratory tract infection signs and symptoms followed by a rapid progression to signs of more severe respiratory distress and fever. Abdominal signs such as distension can also present. Of important note, the right lung is involved in 65% of the cases and is often accompanied by a pleural effusion. Therefore, the CXR findings alone should serve as a good clue to keep your "Staph" on your right side.

221) B) This is a classic description of staphylococcal scalded skin syndrome. The "clear and shiny areas of denuding" is "Nikolsky sign", where areas of the epidermis will separate with minor force or gentle stroking of the skin. The description of crusted lesions around the mouth and nose is another tip off that *Staph* is the guilty party. Remember that erythema multiforme usually involves mucous membranes and would be described as lesions *in* but not around the mouth. Easily remembered as erythema multiORALforme.

---

16 Which would include you, the treating physician.

222) B) The isolation of *Mycobacterium avium* complex would be most suggestive of AIDS in this HIV-positive child. The vignette represents the classic presentation and *is more common in HIV-positive patients who have not received appropriate antiretroviral therapy, which is quite possible in this child whose management is unknown.*

By the way, it is diagnosed via isolation in the blood, bone marrow, or other tissue. *Isolation from stool does not necessarily confirm the diagnosis.* Therefore, watch out for trick questions leading you down that path to the wrong pathogen or wrong diagnostic test.

223) C) This is a fairly straightforward clinical description of an osteomyelitis. The most common cause of osteomyelitis is *Staph aureus*. The absence of swelling or effusion on the knee makes septic arthritis unlikely.

224) E) Fecal H. pylori antigen, endoscopy with biopsy, and urease breath test would all be valid tests to establish the eradication of H. pylori following treatment.

H. Pylori IgG would only be helpful to establish if a patient had or has disease making it only useful in research studies.

If the question had asked for the *preferred noninvasive test* the answer would have been fecal H. pylori antigen

225) C) All childcare and nursery school contacts during the previous 7 days would require chemoprophylaxis. Since this child was exposed 5 days ago chemoprophylaxis for the child is indicated. However since the parents did not have close contact with the index case they will not need chemoprophylaxis.

226) C) Patients with Hepatitis C, genotype 1 do not respond to treatment as well as other genotypes. However they do respond and therefore should be treated.

Treatment is either with interferon or interferon and ribavirin. Ribavirin monotherapy is ineffective.

227) D) The rash and clinical presentation of a centripedal spread of a papular-vesicular rash preceded by fever is consistent with a diagnosis of varicella or chickenpox.

Direct fluorescent antibody would work off of a sample from the lesion itself and would provide the quickest answer. Viral culture would establish the diagnosis but it would take a long time. Polymerase chain reaction would also establish the diagnosis but is not as widely available as direct fluorescent antibody and therefore would not be the quickest method.

Molecular amplification would be appropriate if the virus cannot be detected by rapid isolation as is the case with varicella. Skin biopsy would be completely inappropriate.

Of course back in the old days varicella / chickenpox was a simple diagnosis made on clinical grounds. However, these are the boards and you are expected to know how to confirm the diagnosis definitively.

228) C) Doxycycline and levofloxacin would both be appropriate for treating a skin infection due to a methicillin resistant Staph aureus infection. However the child is 12 and therefore levofloxacin is not approved for routine use in children younger than 18.

Whenever you are asked a question regarding antibiotic choice and are given the patient's age it is important to not which choices can be eliminated based on the age of the patient.

Methicillin resistant Staph aureus would all be resistant to Amoxicillin/ clavulanic acid, cefdinir and amoxicillin.

229) B) Enzyme immunoassay antigen detection (EIA detection) taken from a nasopharyngeal swab would be the most appropriate rapid test for influenza virus. Polymerase chain reaction and viral cultures would both be appropriate but not rapid. EIA detection would be more helpful in the acute setting and direct fluorescent antibody testing would not be the correct test for acute diagnosis of influenza.

230) D) The least effective antibiotic in treating Listeria is cefotaxime. This is because **Listeria is always resistant to cephalosporins.**

---

231) C) Latent CMV infection reactivates if the donor *or* recipient is seropositive. Reactivation often results in severe disease including pneumonitis.

232) C) Changing the diapers or handling the child's laundry is okay with the caveat that washing hands with soap and warm water is done.

However the mother should not sleep in the same bed as the child, no kissing on or near the child's mouth, and no sharing towels or washcloths with the child.

This all stems from the correct assumption that any child younger than 3 is secreting CMV virus in their urine and saliva.

233) D) Both enzyme immunoassay (EIA) and immunofluorescent antibody (IFA) are appropriate tests for confirming the diagnosis of cat scratch disease. Only EIA was among the listed choices and would be the correct answer. .

Antigen skin testing is no longer recommended. Polymerase chain reaction is reliable but not widely available.

234) C) The diagnostic test of choice for rabies is reverse transcriptase-polymerase chain reaction.

Prior rabies immunization does not induce CSF antibody to the virus. Therefore the presence of high CSF antibody titers in the CSF supports the diagnosis of clinical disease.

Clearly the presence of high CSF titers cannot confirm previous disease since previous disease would mean death.

Around 20% of cases many have no documented history of exposure.

235) E) The appropriate treatment for a bite from an animal that could be a carrier of rabies would be a combination of passive and active immunization. This would consist of infiltrating the wound with rabies immunoglobulin. This would be followed by providing HDCV the day the wound was inflicted and then on days 3, 7, 14 and 28.

236) E) While one could argue that A "I am sorry I have to read the question again" is correct it would not be the best answer. You would have to read the question and more importantly write down what each serum marker means in words.

For example:
HBsAb = Hepatitis B Surface antibody.
HBsAg = Hepatitis B Surface antigen
HBcAb total = Hepatitis B core antibody (total IgG and Ig M)
HBcAb IgM = Hepatitis B core antibody acute phase

This makes it much easier to interpret. In this case without the IgM being elevated or the total core antigen being elevated there is no evidence of previous disease or current disease.

The presence of surface antigen supports immunity due to vaccination, which is the correct answer.

237) A) While one could argue that choice E is correct which spells out "Help me I have no idea what the answer is" would be correct, it isn't if you think this through.

If you are asked a question regarding the "replication rate" or "infectivity" of hepatitis B, then you are dealing with the e antigen.

You are either dealing with:
HBeAb (antibody) or HBeAg (antigen). Clearly a low rate of replication or infectivity would be associated with a high HBeAb (antibody) level.

Sonowyouknowhowtoansweranddecodewhatseemedlikeadifficultquestion =
"So know you know how to answer and decode what seemed like a difficult question".

Metabolic

238) D) Although patients with Wolman's disease have elevated total body triglyceride levels and cholesterol levels, these are deposited in body tissue and the serum levels remain normal.

239) 1) (D)
2) (A)
3) (C)
4) (B)

PKU is associated with "mousy odor" urine whatever that is. You won't have to actually smell the urine just identify the association.

Urine smelling like sweaty sox is associated with isovaleric acidemia.

Infants with maple syrup urine disease can present with hypertonia and tachypneic during first week of life.

Dark urine is associated with alcaptonuria.

240) 1) (D)
2) (D)
3) (A)
4) (D)
5) (C)
6) (B)

For #2, Both Menkes Kinky hair syndrome and Wilson Disease are associated with low serum copper levels and ceruloplasmin levels. Therefore "neither" is associated with elevated serum levels. Both disorders involve disruption of copper metabolism. In both cases serum ceruloplasmin levels are elevated and serum copper levels are low. However, total body copper levels are high and are deposited in body tissue in both cases. Only Wilson's disease results in hepatic failure. There is no specific treatment of Menkes kinky hair syndrome (insert your own hair style joke). Treatment for Wilson's disease is D-penicillamine, not penicillin, so remember to read the question carefully.

241) E) Both hereditary fructose intolerance and galactosemia present with vomiting, irritability, and hepatomegaly. Once again, timing is everything. The patient in this question is only 3 weeks old and has been "breast fed". This is the key to the answer and the reason galactosemia is the correct answer.[17]

In addition to seizures, hypoglycemia and cataracts can also be a part of the initial presentation. Elimination of galactose from the diet reverses the clinical manifestations, including the cataracts.

Infants with galactosemia are also vulnerable to gram negative sepsis.

242) D) Elevated homocysteine levels are a known risk factor for cardiovascular disease. The mechanism of action is felt to be via damage to the vascular endothelium. Therefore, children with homocystinuria are at increased risk for a cerebral vascular accident. Treatment is aimed at reducing serum homocysteine levels. Sometimes "pyridoxine"[18] supplementation can reduce homocysteine levels; therefore, homocystinuria is the one metabolic disorder that can sometimes be treated with vitamins. This would be a fair question on the exam.

People with Pompe (Pompous) disease have big heads and egos but not necessarily prone to cerebral vascular accidents.

243) C) The key to getting the question correct is noting the symptoms began **after** breast-feeding stopped and commercial formula and other food sources were introduced. Hereditary fructose intolerance is due to the deficiency of the enzyme 1, 6-biphosphate aldolase. I wouldn't waste time memorizing this; however, it does pay to know the clinical manifestations. The presentation is of an otherwise healthy newborn that after the introduction of feedings becomes symptomatic. Symptoms can include jaundice, hepatomegaly, vomiting, irritability, lethargy, and even coma. Lab findings include hypoglycemia and the presence of **reducing substances** in the urine during an episode.

The symptoms resemble galactosemia, but the timing is wrong for that. Galactosemia would present earlier on and would occur with breast-feeding.

---

[17] Deficiency of uridylyl transferase.
[18] Vitamin B6

244) C) The physical findings in this patient are consistent with Reiter syndrome, best remembered as someone who can't see, can't climb a tree and can't pee, thus you could expect that he would also be complaining of dysuria as a result of urethritis.

245) D) Elevated creatinine phosphokinase concentrations would be consistent with a diagnosis of dermatomyositis.

246) E) Of all the conditions listed soy milk would be most appropriate for a patient with galactosemia. Infants with galactosemia cannot convert galactose to glucose. Therefore soy formula would be most appropriate. Infants with cow milk allergy or allergic colitis cannot tolerate soy formula due to cross reactivity.

247) B) The combination of blunted growth and development along with hypotonia, hepatosplenomegaly and a cherry red spot makes for a diagnosis of Niemann Pick disease. By the way Tay Sachs does not present with hepatosplenomegaly.

Musculoskeletal

248) C) That is because the combination of recent URI, the ability to elicit some passive movement, low WBC and ESR with only "fluid" being found on ultrasound all suggest toxic synovitis which is self limited requiring no other intervention or treatment.

249) D) Since this is "internal tibial torsion", it should resolve by school age without any intervention in the vast majority of cases.

250) C) The goal in treatment is to extend the shoulders and minimize the overlap of the fracture fragments. These fractures heal nicely within 6 weeks, and complications such as Erb palsy or pneumothorax are very rare.

251) E) **Osteoporosis** is what is being described in the clinical vignette, i.e., fragility of the skeletal system and a susceptibility to long bone fractures from mild or inconsequential trauma. *Osteogenesis imperfecta (OI) is the most common genetic cause of osteoporosis.*

In **achondrogenesis** you would see a severe lack of skeletal development, which is typically detected in utero or after a miscarriage.

Fibrochondrogenesis is extremely rare, even on the boards, and has features that are not described in the vignette. For those who are actually interested in what these features are, please see the footnote.[19]

Very short limbs, a short neck, and a long, narrow thorax characterize **thanatophoric dysplasia**; also, a large head with midfacial hypoplasia is dominant. These features were not described in the vignette; therefore, this would not be the best choice.

Juvenile osteochondroses are a group of disorders in which the main features are noninflammatory arthropathies. It would not account for the clinical picture described.

Trifecta imperfecta would be various broken bones secondary to having recommended the horse that came in last to the wrong people.

---

[19] So you are the one person who is actually reading this. Oh well, here it is: The face of someone with fibrochondrogenesis is distinctive and characterized by protuberant eyes, flat midface, a flat, small nose with anteverted nares, and a small mouth with a long upper lip. Cleft palate, micrognathia, and bifid tongue can occur. The limbs show marked shortness of all segments, with relatively normal hands and feet. Now get back to doing real studying.

252) E) These findings are consistent with "nursemaid's elbow", a common injury in toddlers. There is often a history of a caretaker pulling on the arm, perhaps as the child steps off a curb or in various other situations. Watch out while swinging your child around in windmill fashion.

There is no evidence of an infection in the vignette, and radiologic studies are rarely helpful in making the diagnosis. Supinating the forearm while the elbow is flexed is curative and diagnostic; it is one of the most dramatic results in pediatrics.

This condition can reoccurs as a result of an injured, stretched joint capsule., particularly if the parents wait to obtain medical treatment

253) D) A curvature greater than 40 degrees would require surgical intervention to halt further progression and to correct the existing deformity.

For curvature greater than **15-20 degrees, bracing would be indicated to halt progression in a child that is still growing and has not reached full growth potential.** Therefore, watch for inclusion of information that would tell you what stage a teen is in.

For example, a girl who has had menses 2 years prior will probably have little growth potential and will simply need to be observed.

Less than 15-20 degrees would require no intervention.

254) D) Pain described just below the knee over the tibial tubercle in an active adolescent in the absence of other physical findings and history is Osgood-Schlatter.

Osgood-Schlatter is due to microfracture of the proximal tibial epiphysis where the patellar tendon inserts.

In the past rest was the treatment of choice. Since the risk of evulsion is so small removal from sports is no longer recommended. The new recommendation is to play through. Physical activity is limited only if the pain gets severe. Ice and pain management is usually prescribed

With *patellar dislocation* there would be more pain noted, especially with palpation of the patella.

Osteochondritis dissecans occurs when the bone adjacent to the cartilage becomes avascular and separates from the underlying bone. The *knee pain is vague.* If the boy had *osteochondritis dissecans* he would probably have an effusion with palpation of the affected area when his knee is in a flexed position. In addition, the pain is "activity–related," with swelling and "catching and locking" of the knee.

255) D) The loss of physical function in the absence of organic illness suggests a diagnosis of **"conversion disorder or reaction"**. Additional history is needed to make this psychiatric diagnosis of exclusion. It is via a good history that the "precipitating" environmental event will often be uncovered.

The elicitation of deep tendon reflexes in a paralyzed leg in this case is the key to the correct answer. Another example of a conversion reaction might be *hysterical blindness* with normal pupillary response to light. Being cognizant of these classic presentations will help you "convert" an incorrect answer to a correct one.

256) B) After one year of age the development of blood vessels that extend from the metaphysis to the epiphysis disappear. After that point the risk of both osteomyelitis and septic arthritis developing the same area is reduced.

257) C) Clubfoot would present with the inability to dorsiflex the foot which is not seen with metatarsus adductus.

258) A) Scoliosis is defined as a spinal curvature on a **posterior-anterior** x-ray, greater **than 10 degrees.**

259) A) The absence of dystrophin results in muscle sarcolemma instability. This leads to membrane instability which leads to muscle damage and poor muscle function.

260) B) Mothers of an isolated case of Duchenne muscular dystrophy where there is no prior family history and the molecular genetic studies in the patient are negative is closest to 10%

Why you might ask? The answer is, this is due to a germline mosaicism. However that is not what you might be tested on. The 10% recurrence risk is something you might be tested on.

261) A) Congenital talipes equinovarus or club foot is best diagnosed cribside by physical examination.

262) D) This should be an easy question. You would not want to correct club foot when the child begins to walk. Let's face it that might impede the child's ability to learn to walk.

Just prior to entering school would be a bad time to correct a foot deformity that prevented a child from walking. During pubertal development teens have enough problems looking like a microphone stand with a head, without having had a lifetime of walking on club feet. Once the growth plate fuses, adult height has been reached. Damage to self image might be quite impressive at that point.

Neonatology

263) D) Given the SGA status, the best explanation for the jitteriness and the tachypnea is hypoglycemia. There is nothing in the clinical history to suggest asphyxia and bilateral ankle clonus is normal in a newborn. (Despite the perfect clonus rhythm quitting at this point is too risky; you may want to stay in touch and track his career though.) Likewise, sepsis is not likely, especially if IV D10 2-3 mg/kg clears up the problem.

264) D) Ampicillin and Gentamicin still remain the optimal combination in the NICU setting to provide coverage for the most common organisms causing neonatal sepsis. They have minimal toxicity and adequate CSF penetration.

The other possibility among the choices would be ampicillin and cefotaxime However this regimen has resulted in outbreaks of sepsis due to drug resistant organisms.

265) B) It is partially water soluble and therefore less reliant on bile acid and micelle formation. It is also broken down more effectively by lipase. Biliary secretion is hampered by chloride channel abnormalities in CF patients. Remember CF patients have difficulty with exocrine function in general.

266) B) You might be tempted to pick C, but that is usually part of the history and only raises suspicions of choanal atresia, but does not confirm it. The pureed sea conch is for recreational purposes only after you have passed the exam.

267a) B) This is clearly a congenital infection and given the finding of cerebral calcifications you should easily have narrowed your choices down to A and B. However, "retinal irritation" implies chorioretinitis, which is consistent with congenital CMV. Notice that the question did not specify periventricular or diffuse calcifications; therefore, you need to know other factors that distinguish congenital CMV from toxoplasmosis. Retinal hemorrhages which are associated with child abuse would not be described as "retinal irritation".

267b) D) CMV is best diagnosed with a urine culture.

268) 1) (B)
2) (D)
3) (A)
4) (C)
5) (E)

These are the ages when the reflexes listed can be expected to disappear under normal conditions.

The palmar grasp disappears at 4 months.

The plantar grasp disappears at 9 months.

Automatic stepping stops at 2 months.

The moro reflex disappears at 6 months.

The money grasp reflex actually accelerates upon law school graduation, making this a very tricky question.

269) 1) (A)
2) (C)

Transient myasthenia gravis is due to maternal antibody and is self limited thus the descriptive name for the disease. Both forms of myasthenia gravis are diagnosed with a positive Tensilon® test.

270) E) Diabetic mothers have a high incidence of polyhydramnios, pre-eclampsia, and pyelonephritis. Infants of diabetic mothers are at increased risk for congenital anomalies, persistent pulmonary hypertension,[20] and polycythemia. **They are not at increased risk for hypercalcemia.**

---

[20] Due to increased smooth muscle in the pulmonary arteries.

271) D) The history is suggestive of a ductal-dependent congenital heart disease since the onset of symptoms coincides with the closure of the PDA and supplemental oxygen is of no help. Therefore, the most important next step would be to start IV prostaglandins to maintain a patent ductus. Since there is no evidence of respiratory distress, establishing an airway is not necessary. Indomethacin would worsen the problem by closing the duct. Cardiac echo is merely diagnostic and would not be the most appropriate next step.

272) E) Persistent bilious vomiting in a newborn is suggestive of obstruction, and therefore abdominal x-ray would be the next step in order to establish a diagnosis and implement emergency surgical intervention.

If an obstruction were documented on the x-ray then additional studies such as ultrasound might be useful in locating the obstruction. Up to two-thirds of infants with bilious vomiting in the first 72 hours of life have idiopathic vomiting that is benign and resolves.

273) A) Serologic test for syphilis (STS) is usually done at the time of delivery, and congenital syphilis does not produce the findings in this infant. Developmental assessment to approximate the extent of this developmental delay, TORCH titers to confirm the etiology of the intrauterine infection, and evaluation of visual acuity are all-important in this patient. In addition, x-ray studies may reveal intracranial calcifications that, if distributed throughout the brain, would be more consistent with toxoplasma infection than CMV infection.

274) A) Although not specifically stated, *diffuse* intracranial calcifications are consistent with a diagnosis of congenital *toxoplasmosis*.

Treatment with a combination of pyrimethamine and sulfadiazine with folinic acid (leucovorin calcium) to minimize hematological toxicity is the recommended treatment for toxoplasmosis. The potential hematological toxicity is due to pyrimethamine being a potent *folic acid* antagonist.

CBC differential and platelets are indicated once or twice weekly during therapy. Corticosteroids would be indicated for chorioretinitis.

Folic acid is incorrect; make sure you choose folinic acid which is the correct answer.

275) E) The greatest risk factor for hepatitis B in children is perinatal exposure to a hepatitis surface antigen-positive mother. Of all the choices listed, a mother who is a drug user would be at greatest risk for contracting hepatitis B.

A mother from a western European country such as Lichtenstein would not be at high risk. Worldwide, the areas of highest prevalence of HBV infection are sub-Saharan Africa, China, and parts of the Middle East, the Amazon basin, and the Pacific Islands. In addition, the Eskimo population in Alaska has the highest prevalence rate.

276) B) The mention of a breech delivery and the fact that the rash is limited to the buttocks is not random. With the breech presentation it is the buttocks that would have been exposed to the birth canal for the longest period of time and therefore it would be an infection contracted during the birth process.

A vesicular lesion contracted during the birth process could very well be due to exposure to herpes; thus, the most likely diagnosis is herpes simplex neonatorum. Even though they note that the mother's history is negative for herpes does not rule out the possibility of genital herpes at the time of delivery. Of all the choices, this is the most ominous and would require immediate hospitalization to prevent systemic spread.

Indurated subcutaneous plaques on the buttocks and lower back would be consistent with subcutaneous fat necrosis, which is a benign self-limited disorder seen in healthy newborns.

Pigmented macules would be consistent with transient neonatal pustular melanosis, a benign eruption often seen at birth.

Flat bluish discoloration over the posterior spine and buttocks would be a mongolian spot and not ominous at all.

277) E) Since the physical findings and the clinical condition are both normal, this would be classified as "*peripheral cyanosis*" or "*acrocyanosis*" and all that would be required would be placement under a radiant warmer; that in and of itself would solve the problem. Had they described *central cyanosis* along with other signs, it would entail an entirely different workup.

278) D) The non-stress test measures fetal heart rate reactivity in response to spontaneous fetal movements. It therefore measures fetal autonomic nervous system integrity. At around 29 weeks and later gestation when the baby moves, the HR should increase at least 15 beats above baseline for 15 seconds or more. This indicates normal activity.

The non stress test does not measure fetal maturity.

279) C) Abdominal distension past the first 48 hours would be consistent with a lower bowel obstruction requiring a contrast enema to make the diagnosis.

280) C) Neonatal mastitis would present with unilateral enlargement, erythema, and tenderness. Therefore IV antibiotics won't be indicated.

Since the genitalia appear normal and there are no other abnormalities described, an endocrinological workup including skull x-ray would not be indicated.

Bilateral breast hypertrophy is a common finding in newborns. It is secondary to elevated estrogen levels late in pregnancy and will resolve spontaneously. The milky discharge is also a common finding and is known as "witch's milk".

An old wives' tale recommends squeezing the breasts to alleviate the problem. This may actually exacerbate the condition and is ill advised, especially in the presence of a freaked-out father. Reassurance is the order of the day in this case.

Perhaps a review father's medication and diet would be in order but this would probably not be the next most appropriate step.

281) E) With this question some of the systematic steps suggested for *all* questions would come in handy to reason this out. Since this question contains all of the numbers needed to calculate the anion gap that should be the first step.

In this case the anion gap is 25 (sodium minus chloride minus the bicarb). Since the anion gap is normally in the 12-16 range, in this case we are dealing with an *increased anion gap.*

The question is now reduced to "Which of the following diagnoses are consistent with an elevated anion gap?" and you would correctly identify the one disease with a metabolic acidosis and an elevated anion gap, which is maple syrup urine disease.

Since distal and proximal renal tubular acidoses are distinguished from each other by the *urine pH* and this information is not provided, you can almost eliminate these choices. But what allows you to eliminate these choices with certainty is the fact that the "loss of bicarb is compensated with the retention of chloride," resulting in a normal anion gap with both renal tubular acidoses.

With the PCO_2 of 28, there is clear evidence of an attempt at respiratory compensation for the acidosis. Therefore, there is no respiratory failure. Polycystic kidney disease does not cause metabolic acidosis.

282) E) "To suck mec or not to suck mec" is one of the proverbial question that plagues residents and neonatologist through the ages.

Unfortunately the answer and rationale changes with the wind , and if you do not keep up, the mec will hit the fan.

Current recommendations take into account the infant's clinical status rather than the appearance of the mec itself.

Current recommendation do not take into consider the consistency of the meconium. Endotracheal intubation and suction would bei indicated if the infant is not vigorous, needs positive pressure ventilation or develops respiratory distress after the initial assessment.

The infant in the vignette is vigorous after 1 minute , therefore no resuscitation is indicated despite the thick meconium.

283) B) A child who is born at 32 weeks gestation would be 8 weeks behind. Therefore, the developmental milestones should be at 4 months, which would be consistent with the milestones described in choice B.

284) D) Given that the patient is asymptomatic, the rash is classic for *erythema toxicum.* The anxiety is misguided since this is a harmless, self-limited rash that appears within the first 1-2 days of life and usually disappears spontaneously within days.

285) D) All trisomies, including Trisomy 13, 18, and 21, are associated with a *decreased* alpha-fetoprotein level. Elevated levels are associated with neural tube defects, multiple gestations, and defects in the abdominal wall (bladder exstrophy and omphalocele).

286) A) Dietary protein intolerance is a *non* IgE mediated food hypersensitivity to egg, soy and milk proteins. It can present with heme positive stools, vomiting , and diarrhea and in severe cases failure to thrive.

It typically occurs during the first year of life.

287) B) Hypochloremic, hypokalemic, metabolic alkalosis would be expected in pyloric stenosis. Because of the persistent projective vomiting seen in pyloric stenosis, normal bicarb production is not buffered by hydrogen produced in the stomach. In addition due to volume contraction triggers increased proximal tubular reabsorption of bicarbonate. This leads to metabolic *alkalosis.*

Chloride is lost through persistent emesis and the lack of hydrogen ions results in enhanced excretion of potassium leading to hypokalemia.

Although congenital adrenal hyperplasia can lead to electrolyte disturbances, *hyper*kalemia would be the result.

Neurology

288) D) Todd postictal paralysis, hemiparetic seizures, a subdural hemorrhage and hypoglycemia could each explain acute lateralized weakness.

However hypocalcemia would not result in acute lateralized weakness.

289) Part 1: E)

This is a classic history of infantile botulism. Although it classically occurs with ingestion of honey, on the boards and in the real world there will rarely be a history of honey ingestion or any other food. That would suggest a diagnosis of infantile botulism. This lack of history is especially true on the boards.

Only 10-25% of cases are related to honey, cases not related to honey are usually in rural areas where there is a lot of soil exposure.

Part 2: E)

Treatment of infantile botulism is **primarily** supportive.

Antibiotics are not indicated. Gentamicin would particularly be contraindicated since it is associated with neurotoxicity

While one could argue that this question belongs in the ID section, doing so would tip the answer too easily.

290) A) Diazepam (rectal valium) has been found effective when given by parents at the onset of fever. Unfortunately, giving antipyretics alone is rarely effective in preventing febrile seizures, especially when choosing the correct answer on the boards. No intervention is needed unless there are several recurrences during the year and parental anxiety and concern becomes an important factor.

While giving antipyretics at the onset of fever would be appropriate of the choices listed it would not be the best way to prevent febrile seizures.

291) A) This is a classic description of **tuberous sclerosis**. Head CT would reveal the "tubers" projecting into the ventricles. The hypopigmented patches are likely to be ash leaf spots and the bump would be a sebaceous adenoma.

292) 1) (C)
2) (B)
3) (A)
4) (D)

Both infantile botulism and myasthenia gravis can involve the eyes.

Only myasthenia gravis would present with a progressive onset. Infantile botulism would present with a more acute clinical picture.

Myasthenia gravis is managed but not cured.

Infantile botulism only requires supportive care but this would be curative. The patient should have no residual effects.

Neither myasthenia gravis nor infantile botulism is prevented with immunization.

293) 1) (B)
2) (C)
3) (A)

A cough that is exaggerated by sneezing, coughing, or straining would suggest the increased intracranial pressure associated with a headache due to a space-occupying or **structural headache**.

Cyclic vomiting and recurrent abdominal pain also are frequently considered **migraine variants**. **Tension headaches** are due to muscle tension or muscle contraction. Tension headaches are often described as feeling like a band around the head or occasionally as pain in the neck or shoulders

294) A) With the focal findings of "mild lower extremity hyperreflexia" coupled with the early morning vomiting and headaches, the past history of migraine headaches would not be a factor in managing this patient at this time.

An MRI of the head to rule out a space-occupying lesion like a tumor is the most appropriate next step.

295) A) The average head circumference of a full-term infant at birth measures 34–35 cm; and this would be the definition of a normocephalic full term.

Therefore a head circumference of 39 cm in a full term newborn would represent macrocephaly. No other conclusions can be drawn given the information provided in the question.

296) C) When presented with a neonatal seizure, don't reflexively go down the well-trodden path of ischemic encephalopathy. The EEG pattern described is typical of **pyridoxine dependency**, a rare autosomal recessive disorder.

297) E) The combination of an infant with "descending paralysis"[21] and "constipation" makes for the classic presentation of infantile botulism.

Myasthenia gravis would not be of sudden onset, and **Werdnig-Hoffman** disease affects the anterior horn cells and presents with generalized muscle weakness and the sparing of the *extraocular muscles.*

298) D) The combination of diplopia, tinnitus and vertigo in a context of intermittent occipital headaches is a classic description of basilar-type migraine headaches. Patients are fine in between episodes and the neurological exam in unremarkable.

---

[21] Remember to write what is being described in the margins.

299) C) Regular sleep, exercise, biofeedback and stress management all are recognized as methods to reduce the frequency and severity of migraine headaches.

However an elimination diet which refers to the wholesale elimination of a list of foods is not recommended. It is more prudent to make a list of foods which can potentially trigger a migraine headache and note if there is a temporal relationship.

300) C) This is a classic description of medication overuse headaches which were previously known as rebound headaches. This is a result of the overuse of analgesics which shut down the bodies own endogenous response to headaches. Analgesics should not be used more than a couple of times per week.

If more pain management is required then *prophylactic migraine medications* would be indicated including:

Tricyclic antidepressants such as amitriptyline
Calcium channel blockers
Beta blockers
Anticonvulsants

Sumatriptan although not noted as one of the medications being used to treat the headache, would not be considered prophylactic. Therefore it would not be one of the correct choices if you were asked how to manage this patient.

301) D) The clinical vignette is classic for **absence seizures**. The EEG pattern for absence seizures would be a 3 per second generalize spike and wave pattern.

The appropriate treatment would be ethosuximide, lamotrigine or valproate.

Carbamazepine makes absence seizures worse.

This can be remembered by picturing somebody with a petit mal seizure in the middle an amusement park bumper car park getting "bammed by a car" (carbamazepine)

The clinical description is not consistent with ADHD and therefore neither atomoxetine nor methylphenidate would be appropriate treatment options.

302) B) The ketogenic diet (high fat low carbohydrate) has been shown to be effective in managing infantile spasms. In addition adrenocorticotropic (ACTH) hormone, valproic acid and topiramate are all considered first line treatment of infantile spasms.

Nutrition

303) B) Human milk does provide passive immunity via IgA. Breast-feeding provides complete nutrition for growth, development, and hydration during the first 6 months of life thus the recommendation by the APA for **exclusive breast feeding during the first 6 months of life.**

It is true that family support is crucial for breast-feeding success. However health care providers including pediatricians have actually been one of the barriers to successful breast-feeding by not providing adequate resources and information.

304) C) Breast milk is known to contain IgA, immunomodulating agents to enhance the breast-feeding infants own immune system, anti-inflammatory agents, and anti-microbial agents.

However choice C, IgG would be incorrect since IgG is *not* present in breast milk.

305)
1) (B)
2) (E)
3) (A)
4) (D)
5) (C)

Retinol deficiency is the leading cause of blindness worldwide.

Tocopherol deficiency is associated with hemolytic anemia.

Deficiency of phylloquinone, or vitamin K is associated with hemorrhagic disease of the newborn.

Thiamine deficiency is associated with peripheral paralysis and muscle weakness.

Riboflavin deficiency is associated with angular stomatitis and seborrheic dermatitis.

306) 1) (C)
2) (B)
3) (A)

Tocopherol which is also known as vitamin E can result in liver toxicity.

Niacin also known as vitamin B_3 can result in vasodilation if taken in toxic doses.

Ascorbic acid or vitamin C taken in excessive dosages can lead to nephrocalcinosis.

307) E) Changing eating habits in the long term would be the most difficult to implement and is associated with poor long term compliance.

The most effective way to implement long-term diet changes would be to coordinate the plan in conjunction with the whole family.

308) E) If you are managing a 36 hour newborn with persistent bilious vomiting ruling out a surgical emergency such as midgut volvulus must be the first priority.

The abdominal film would therefore be the *most appropriate* next step in managing this patient. This could be a surgical emergency, which would need to be done immediately.

If indicated, a sepsis workup can be done after the x-ray. This would be the MOST appropriate next step. *In many cases, the bilious vomiting is not due to an obstruction and is only a transient problem requiring no intervention however initially this would not be known.*

309) D) Calciferol is another name for vitamin D. **Vitamin D deficiency** can result in high serum phosphatase levels, infantile tetany, poor growth and osteomalacia.

Calciferol regulates the absorption and deposition of calcium and phosphorus. High serum phosphatase levels can appear prior to the bone deformities seen with rickets.

However calciferol or vitamin D deficiency does not result in pharyngeal ulcers.

310)   B)   Niacin (Vitamin B₃) deficiency can result in pellagra, which manifests as GI distress, dementia, and skin manifestations, including rash.

Xerophthalmia is associated with vitamin A (retinol) deficiency, not niacin deficiency.

311)   E)   Foods containing oats, barley, rye, and wheat must be substituted with foods containing *corn and rice*. This can be best remembered with the mnemonic "**B**eware **of R**otten **W**heat" to remember that it is barley, oats, rye, and wheat that should be avoided in celiac disease.

You could add that **C**orn is **OC**ay

312)   D)   The clinical description is of scurvy which is seen in infants fed evaporated milk without supplementation. The irritability, generalized tenderness (the explanation for the child being irritable and not wanting to be touched), petechiae, gum swelling are all consistent with vitamin C (ascorbic acid) deficiency.

The x-ray findings, thinning of the cortices, ground glass appearance of the bones and calcified cartilage at the metaphysis are also consistent with scurvy.

The most appropriate treatment would be ascorbic acid supplementation.

313)   D   Joint aches, headache and lethargy are all consistent with retinol or vitamin A toxicity. The increased opening pressure on LP would be consistent with this diagnosis and the absence of white blood cells in an atraumatic tap (absence of red blood cells) would rule out aseptic meningitis.

There is nothing in the history to suggest trauma or migraine headaches. Retinol deficiency would not present with these symptoms.

314)   A)   The skin color, prematurity and exclusive breast feeding places this child at risk for vitamin D deficiency and the clinical picture of rickets.

There is nothing to suggest a diagnosis of vitamin, E, D or A deficiency. Likewise there is nothing to suggest a diagnosis of iron deficiency or cystic fibrosis.

315)   E)   Despite the urban medical myth of the BRATT diet the appropriate treatment if tolerated is oral rehydration and a regular diet to assure that the child is getting adequate nutrition.

The only restriction would be fluids containing a high concentration of sugar.

316)   D)   If you remember the adage "if the gut works use it" this is an easy question. Since the presence of absence of air fluid levels will be critical in knowing if the gut isn't working

Enteral feeding is always preferred especially since it is known to actually decrease inflammation and stimulate the production of digestive enzymes. Parenteral feedings should be avoided since it lacks these advantages plus there is the added risk of line infection and other complications.

317)   D)   Home prepared foods do not decrease the risk of food allergies. Standard bottled vegetables may contain more sugar and salt than an infant can tolerate. Honey should never be given to an infant during the first year of life.

Home prepared products should be pureed and *can be frozen and used later.*

Exclusive breastfeeding during the first 6 months has been shown to decrease the risk of allergies and is advocated by the AAP.

Pharmacology

318) E) St. John's wort can decrease the efficacy of oral contraceptive pills by inducing the cytochrome P-450 pathway speeding up the elimination of oral contraceptive pills and decreasing its bioavailability .

319) A) Echinacea is contraindicated in patients taking immunosuppressant medications. Just note this it will come in handy on the exam.

320) B) Ginseng can interact with oral hypoglycemic agents, oral anticoagulants, antiplatelet agents as well as corticosteroids.

321) B) The fact that it is BID is not really relevant. What is relevant is that a steady state (no not Maryland) is achieved in 5 days (5 twenty-four hour periods) and that it takes 5 half lives to reach a steady state. Therefore, the half-life is closest to one day, which is 24 hours.

322) D) Hypertension does not alter the serum levels of medications. All of the other choices have the potential to alter serum albumin levels, and anything that alters serum albumin alters the effectiveness of a variety of medications. Juvenile polyps reduce the serum albumin level because of general protein loss.

Preventive

323) D) Children older than 2-1/2 need to receive no more than 35% of their caloric intake from fat. All the other choices are incorrect. Screening should be started at 2 not 1. If family history alone were used as a parameter in choosing whom to screen, many children with hypercholesterolemia would be missed. Also, hypercholesteremia can have many causes such as nephrotic syndrome and hypothyroidism. It is a low HDL, which is a worrisome sign in both children and adults. The opposite is true with LDL, that is, a low LDL is a good sign and a high LDL is a worrisome sign.

324) A) Sideroblastic anemia is the only listed disorder not associated with hyperlipidemia.

325) C) Methanol, when abused, is associated with blindness. Ethanol, administered under medical supervision, is the antidote. However, it is not associated with hyperlipidemia.

326) D) A previous diagnosis of pertussis is difficult to confirm. Administering any pertussis vaccine to someone with a previous history of natural disease *poses no safety concerns.* The duration of protection after infection with B. pertussis is unknown. Therefore Tdap should be administered according to routine recommendations to a 12 year old with a previous history of pertussis.

327) B) Since more than 5 years has elapsed since the most recent dose, a booster is indicated. Children older than 7 should receive the adult strength diphtheria and tetanus toxoid vaccine. Had this child received the booster recommended at 4-1/2 years, then no immunization would be needed at this point.

328) B) Infants **do** normally cry more during the second month; however, colic rarely occurs after the third month. Crying peaks at age 6 weeks, just when the baby starts to smile and the parents smile as well.

Parental fear and anxiety can play a role in colic, e.g., climbing up the entertainment center.[22,23] Infants can of course cry in response to many things besides hunger. Flexion of the arms and legs are not diagnostic of colic. These symptoms can be part of normal crying or be suggestive of a serious gastrointestinal problem such as obstruction.

329) B) Alcohol consumption is the most frequent problem associated with teen accidents and injuries.

330) B) HIV infection would not be a contraindication for the MMR vaccine and neither would a child with ALL in remission. A child with sickle cell disease or otitis media can also receive the vaccine.

Precautions are suggested with thrombocytopenia and for any child who has received immune globulin within the past 3 to 11 months. Therefore, a child with ITP receiving IV IG should not receive the vaccine.

Other contraindications include pregnancy, history of an anaphylactic reaction to neomycin or gelatin, long-term immunosuppressive therapy, and *active* hematological or solid tumors.

331) E) This would be a question that falls under the category of "it looks easier than it is". Logically it would appear that unilateral testicle would be a contraindication to contact sports. However, it is not. Wearing a protective cup may be a good idea, nonetheless.

Acute diarrhea resulting in severe dehydration and fever should be resolved prior to participation in contact sports. Hepatomegaly or splenomegaly could result in a rupture of either organ, and either should be resolved prior to participation.

Any skin lesion, including impetigo that can be spread by direct "contact" would make participation in contact sports contraindicated.

---

[22] Such activities are best done away from the home, and away from law enforcement.
[23] If the infant-crying to father-whining ratio is greater than 2 you should be concerned.

332) C) Suicide is the second leading cause of death among adolescents. While girls attempt suicide more frequently, boys are "more successful," partly because they choose more violent and definitive means. Firearms are the most common method used in "successful" suicide attempts. Only a fraction of all suicide attempts come to medical attention. Television has been shown to increase suicide attempt rates.

333) A) You probably recognize serum gamma glutamyl transferase as one of the liver function tests. An elevated GGT correlates with chronic alcohol abuse, as does an *increased* mean corpuscle volume. Hypoglycemia, metabolic acidosis, and elevated blood alcohol levels all correlate with *acute* alcohol toxicity rather than chronic alcohol abuse.

334) E) There is an association between the use of anabolic steroids and the use of other drugs. Teens who use anabolic steroids are more likely to engage in fighting behavior. Teens who abuse drugs in general are more likely to engage in violent behavior, regardless of gender.

Psychosocial

335) C) Of all the risk factors listed homosexual teens are at the highest risk for suicide.

336) D) The delay of developmental milestones is the main sign of mental retardation. However, marked delays in psychomotor skills in the first year of life is more a feature of more *severe* retardation.

Normal motor development with delayed speech and language abilities in the toddler years is more typical of *moderate* retardation.

On the other hand, **mild** retardation is usually not suspected until after entry into school. Participation in an organized preschool can highlight discrepancies prior to school entry, but they are *most likely* to be diagnosed at school entry.

337) A) Autism has not been associated with trisomy 21. However, all of the other choices listed are associated with autism. Other conditions not listed, which include neurofibromatosis, encephalitis, maternal rubella, and infantile spasms are associated with autism.

338) C) Dyslexia is the *most common* developmental language disorder. It is frequently diagnosed in the 4th grade, when a child is called upon to use the reading skills learned in earlier grades. However, children with high cognitive abilities can sometimes compensate. If there is adequate compensation then the diagnosis often doesn't occur until adulthood, if at all. Autopsies of adults with dyslexia have resulted in the documentation of a possible anatomical basis for the disease.

339) C) A 3-year-old with an otherwise normal history and physical exam who has marked speech delay should be assumed to have a hearing deficit until proven otherwise. Appropriate identification and intervention should be a top priority.

The following table is a rough guideline of red flags by age to keep in mind to determine when a hearing evaluation would be indicated. This is important when presented with a similar history on the exam, and should help you decide when a hearing screen would be the appropriate answer:

Age	Deficit
1 year old	Lack of vocal imitation
1-1/2 year old	The inability to use single words
2 year old	A vocabulary of less than 10 words
3 year old (the patient in the vignette)	A vocabulary of less than 200 words and less than 1/2 their words are understood

340) B) An infant who is older than 6 months but younger than 9 months should be able to babble and transfer an object from one hand to the other. A child less than 9 months old wouldn't be able to hold two objects; likewise they would not be able to lift their bellies off the floor until age 9 months.

Most 18-year-olds can and will babble and transfer a cube from one hand to another; however, one of the objects would have to be an I-Pod ®

341) B) These milestones are most consistent with that of a 2-month-old infant. A child of 2 months should be able to lift his head while lying down.

342) D) Adopted children should be informed when their verbal skills and comprehension are adequate to grasp the information. The topic should be brought up naturally when appropriate, i.e., at the birth of other relatives or friends. The topic should be discussed when the child wishes to, and information appropriate to age and developmental stage should be available. However, it should not be discussed in excess. Discussing the subject when it naturally comes up would be the best way to "normalize" the situation.

343) E) Because of the risk of hepatotoxicity, pemoline should no longer be prescribed for ADHD.

344) E) There is no evidence that any herbal or supplemental medications work in the treatment of ADHD. Likewise there is also no evidence that dyes, preservatives, or sugar in the diet cause or worsens this condition. A multimodal approach including stimulant[24] medication and behavioral interventions is the most successful approach to managing ADHD. Often the results are dramatic; around 70% of kids respond favorably to stimulant medication.

---

[24] And, when contraindicated, other medications.

345) A) This is one of those questions on approach and ethics. Clearly the first choice is the only one that would not alienate the parents and would get them to agree to this important procedure. However surgery cannot wait another 6 months.

346) C) The combination of "ritualistic", "withdrawn" behavior coupled with tantrums at 24 months of age is typical for autism. Autism is also characterized by abnormal language development. Therefore, the correct answer would be abnormal language development. Stranger anxiety would not be an issue since autistic children show lack of closeness to the parents. They would not necessarily distinguish parent from stranger.

347) B) Regarding faces, smiling responsively, laughs, staring at hands for a few seconds, and not responding to a sound or reaching for a toy that is out of reach would be consistent with the developmental milestones of a 2 month old.

348) E) Although some 18-month-olds might know more than 12 words, the use of considerable jargon is normal for a child that age.[25] The use of 2-word sentences would also not be "normal" at this stage; it is a 24-month skill. Therefore, reassurance is the correct answer as is often the case on the exam and in practice.

349) D) **Sexual orientation** is refers to the physical and emotional arousal toward other people. Is the gender, male or female, that a person identifies with?

Sexual orientation is biologically based but is determined by genetic, hormonal and environmental influences

Homosexual teens are at a *higher risk* to drop out than their heterosexual peers.

Sexual orientation is *not a choice* therefor parents should not be told that their children are *free to choose* their sexual orientation.

However sexual behavior and activity are choices teens make.

---

[25] As well as pediatricians at major meetings.

350) D) Vaginal discharge and irritation could be due to physiologic vaginitis. Interest in wearing men's clothing would not be abnormal and neither would reluctance to undress in front of the mother.

However imitation of adult sexual activities would not be expected or normal and would warrant further investigation

351) B) A child with a progressively debilitating illness will be aware of the severity of their condition. The most appropriate option would be to explain to the child consistent with their developmental ability to understand.

352) A) In a family with vulnerable child syndrome, children will develop several symptoms that you are expected to be aware of. Child symptoms include sleep problems, hyperactivity, *underachievement*, and learning difficulties.

They can also engage in risk behaviors that reinforce parental fears, which by definition are unwarranted.

Vulnerable child syndrome is often due to parental failure to understand the connection between the past and current events. Children are typically brought for medical care excessively. It is most important to establish the diagnosis through history and physical exam.

353) B) Peak onset of separation anxiety disorder is middle childhood around age 7-9 the symptoms can persist into childhood and into early adulthood, including difficulty with going away to college.

Children with separation anxiety disorder often have other psychiatric disorders.

Some studies show that it occurs primarily in females, but new studies show prevalence among males.

354) D) It is recommended that children resume regular school attendance without the parent present and without gradual withdrawal of parents.

This might seem to contradict the exposure based cognitive behavioral therapy which emphasizes gradual introduction of fearful situations. However this stage is best done cold turkey because a child's anxiety tends to decrease soon after a parent leaves.

They can then use some of the techniques to reduce anxiety that they were taught during the therapeutic process.

Pulmonary

355) D) Grunting is a common finding in infants who have pneumonia. Persistent cough is a common finding in children *outside the newborn period.* Coughs due to upper respiratory infection are most prominent *at night* and the younger the child is the more likely the cough is due to pneumonia.

356) B) *Malignant hyperpyrexia* or *malignant hyperthermia* is due to a rare life-threatening genetic abnormality of skeletal muscle and is characterized by

- Tachycardia
- Tachypnea,
- Hypermetabolism
- Muscle rigidity,
- Hypercarbia,
- Acidosis,
- Fever

In addition to vapor inhalation anesthetics (*halothane, isoflurane*) it can occur after exposure to depolarizing muscle relaxants such as succinylcholine.

357) E) The most likely diagnosis would be a foreign body aspiration. Keep in mind that on the exam they will rarely describe the precipitating episode. They will usually describe a "sudden onset" of coughing in a mobile toddler and/or localized wheezing, as described in this vignette.

358) E) Asthmatic children should not be discouraged from participating in exercise. *Exercise-induced asthma* can best be prevented with the inhalation of a beta -agonist immediately before exercise. Inhaled albuterol usually affords protection for 4 hours; use of a muffler or cold-weather mask to warm and humidify air before inhalation might help as well, but supplemental oxygen shouldn't be necessary. Inhaled steroids would be a good *preventives long term* measure, but would not be effective immediately prior to exercise.

359) D) There are a few clues here in the question that should make this a simple one to answer correctly. Remember, nothing is mentioned in the question without a reason. A visit to the aunt when the cough started "suddenly" suggests that perhaps the house was not child-proofed and it is therefore possible that the toddler got his hands on something he shouldn't have.

The fact that the child is afebrile, with no history of asthma and no family history of asthma, points away from reactive airway disease or bronchiolitis. The x-ray findings further substantiate this diagnosis.

Psychogenic cough presents as a cough that disappears at night, and this was not the scenario noted in the history.

360) D) Wheezing and expiratory wheeze in a patient who is post op for TE fistula repair makes, tracheomalacia the most likely diagnosis. Tracheomalacia and is often a frequent cause of respiratory distress in a child following surgical repair of a TE fistula post. Tracheomalacia is caused by the collapse of the trachea and larynx and the resultant airway obstruction and wheezing with expiration.

The symptoms described are not consistent with the recurrence of a TE fistula, which would present choking and heavy secretions with feeding.

361) B) Onset of asthma prior to the first year, elevated IgE levels, eosinophilia, and the presence of rhinitis during the first year are all risk factors for asthma persisting past adolescence.

However, recurrent viral illnesses would not be considered to be a risk factor.

Frequently recurrent viral illnesses present during early childhood triggers reactive airways in kids who go on to be diagnosed with asthma. Once the frequency of the viral illnesses decreases, so should the episodes of reactive airway and asthmatic flare-ups. Since the frequency of viral illnesses decreases after adolescence so should clinical asthma.

362) B) Unlike in adults, TB is often "silent" (without coughing or other typical TB symptoms) in children, which makes screening in high-risk groups particularly important. The best way to tell if a child has TB is by obtaining a PPD.

363) C) The key is the "rapid onset". The best explanation for the *rapid* onset of symptoms versus a gradual onset of symptoms would be a pneumothorax.

Pneumothorax occurs in 10%-25% of patients with CF who are older than 10, and the patient in this question would be at risk because he is 15 years old.

364) D) The absence of cough during sleep will almost always be the clue that the cause of the cough is not pulmonary in origin. Therefore, the tic disorder or psychogenic cough is confirmed by the absence of cough during sleep.

Likewise, a "Psychogenic cough" would also be the correct answer if they presented a patient whose cough disappeared at night and they asked for a diagnosis.

365) E) This is a classic description of exercise-induced asthma.

An x-ray is not needed to diagnosis asthmatics in a 14 year old. However if this was a question involving a pre-school aged child an x-ray would be helpful since pulmonary function tests would be unreliable.

When asthma is suspected, pulmonary function testing (PFT) is the best way to confirm the diagnosis. Spirometry pre and post bronchodilator therapy demonstrating revisable airway obstruction is gold standard in diagnosing asthma

366) D) Steroids improve pulmonary function compared with the use of bronchodilators alone with acute asthma. Inhaled anticholinergic agents should not be used routinely since there is no current proof that they provide any benefit.

While in practice it is not uncommon to treat children with fever and a cough during an acute exacerbation with antibiotics it would not be a correct choice on the exam. The fever and cough are most likely due to a viral illness

Some patients, especially those on high dose inhaled steroids do better with a longer course of steroids that require tapering than a shorter course.

367) A) Mild persistent asthma is

· General symptoms greater than 2 times a week
· Night symptoms greater than 2 times a month

Acute exacerbations should be treated with bronchodilators and systemic steroids depending on the severity.

Daily treatment mild persistent asthma is most appropriately treated with

1st Line - inhaled steroids
2nd line – leukotriene modifier if inhaled steroids are not working

Cromolyn and/or theophylline can be used but are not first line treatments

368) D) Chronic use of inhaled steroids has a minimal if any impact on adult height. If "no impact on adult height" were one of the choices it would be correct.

Systemic absorption can be minimized with the use of spacers and mouth rinsing after use.

Chest x-rays in preschool children can be helpful since it is very difficult to perform pulmonary function testing in preschool children. Therefore pulmonary function testing is *not* the most objective measurement of improvement for preschool children.

Children whose asthma is triggered only by viral illness do have moderate persistent asthma.

369) D) African American children are hospitalized *more frequently* than Caucasian children.

Early child care exposure and household "exposure" resulting in frequent viral infections *offers protection from allergies and asthma* at age 7.

However, early child care exposure and household "exposure" resulting in frequent viral infections *have a higher incidence of wheezing before age 2.*

370) D) The incidence of pneumonia is higher in children from lower socioeconomic levels, and in boys more than girls. Fever and cough are hallmark symptoms of pneumonia although clearly not diagnostic. Pneumonia is often diagnosed and treated on clinical grounds and chest x-ray confirmation is not required for treatment. Tachypnea can be a presenting sign but is not required for diagnosis.

Renal

371) B) Autosomal-dominant kidney disease is also known as **adult polycystic disease**. The kidneys are enlarged and show cortical and medullary cysts that are primarily dilated tubules. This can be diagnosed with renal ultrasound, IVP, or CT scan. Of all the choices listed, **renal ultrasound** would be the most appropriate initial step in helping to establish a diagnosis.

372) B) Gross or microscopic hematuria in the absence of any other clinical evidence or diagnostic confirmation may just be due to exercise. Therefore, observation and perhaps an activity log to correlate with the episodes of hematuria would be the most appropriate next step in this patient. Hematuria should resolve within 48 hours when the urine analysis is repeated.

373) A) Each of the conditions listed can result in hypertension with the exception of Bartter's syndrome. **William's syndrome** and **neurofibromatosis** can affect the renal vasculature, resulting in increased renin secretion. Patients with **post strep glomerulonephritis,** for example, can present with hypertension, and **pyelonephritis** can result in hypertension as well.

This is sort of a trick question since Bartter's syndrome **can result in elevated serum renin levels** as well as polyuria. **Hypertension,** however, is not seen in this syndrome.

374) E) Post strep glomerulonephritis typically involves the glomerulus, **not the renal tubules.** Therefore, children with post strep glomerulonephritis have no difficulty concentrating their urine. Children with **sickle cell dis**ease can have the impaired ability to concentrate urine when the disease affects the kidneys. This is called *hyposthenuria*. **Acute tubular necrosis, diabetes insipidus and Barters' syndrome** can also affect the kidney's ability to concentrate urine.

375) B) The most likely diagnosis is *benign proteinuria,* or perhaps orthostatic proteinuria, which is the most common cause of asymptomatic proteinuria in teens. An *AM urine protein / creatinine ratio* is more accurate than a urine dipstick. There is no indication of more severe renal disease or a UTI in the lab or clinical findings described.

376) A) Low serum C_3 levels are seen with membranoproliferative glomerulonephritis, acute post strep glomerulonephritis, and lupus nephritis. However, low serum C_3 is not seen with focal segmental glomerulonephritis.

There is, low serum C_3 is only seen in the early stages of disease in acute post strep glomerulonephritis, up to 8 weeks, and always returns to normal. This helps distinguish acute post strep glomerulonephritis from membranoproliferative glomerulonephritis and lupus nephritis.

377) D) SIADH results in fluid retention and **decreased urine output.** Therefore, it will unlikely result in enuresis. On the other hand, diabetes insipidus would be associated with excessive urine output and could result in enuresis. Sickle cell disease can have an effect on the kidney's ability to concentrate urine. Seizure disorders can result in urinary incontinence, and lumbosacral anomalies could impact bladder tone.

You can remember that SIADH is associated with retention of fluid with low urine output by memorizing it as "Syndrome of I am definitely hydrated".

378) C) Hemolytic uremic syndrome does occur primarily during the summer months and more often in pre-schoolers (ages 6 months to 4 years). It actually occurs more frequently in families of **higher, not lower, socioeconomic status,** possibly due to the types of foods consumed. It is seen more often in the Northern US and Canada, so choice E is incorrect.

Please note that *E. coli,* the causative agent, is not exclusively found in undercooked ground meat; it can also be found in cheese, yogurt, and mayonnaise.

379) B) Struvite stones are associated with urinary tract infections with organisms which contain urease. In fact struvite stones form *only* in the setting of infection.

380) A) Inflammatory bowel disease is associated with increased absorption of oxalate. Therefore this patient most likely has an oxalate stone.

381) E) Increased water intake and low sodium diet are the first line treatments for hematuria and stones due to hypercalciuria.

Thiazide diuretics would be considered a 2nd line treatment not first.

382) C) Hematuria and proteinuria occurring together will always indicate serious renal disease on the boards. This would include a variety of nephritides, Alport syndrome, or post strep glomerulonephritis.

383) A) A diagnosis of congenital nephrotic syndrome is associated with anasarca, low serum thyroid –binding globulin, and low serum transferrin due to these and other protein being lost in the urine.

The kidneys appear hyperechogenic and *large* on ultrasound.

384) E) The most appropriate management would be to repeat the urine analysis since the proteinuria could be transiently associated with the febrile illness.

Other causes of a transient proteinuria which must be factored in include vigorous exercise, dehydration, or stress.

385) A) **Hyper**kalemia is an adverse effect of ACE inhibitors not hypokalemia. The other choices including neutropenia, angioedema, anemia and even dry cough are potential adverse effects of ACE inhibitors in children.

Rheumatology

386) A) It is important to remember that it is **arthritis** which is one of the Major Jones criteria and **arthralgia** one of the minor criteria

Likewise, erythema chronicum migrans is associated with Lyme disease; erythema marginatum is associated with rheumatic fever.

If you had known either of these facts this question is a slam dunk.

387) D) Kawasaki disease is more common in Asian populations and among females. It is more commonly seen in the winter and spring than in the summer and fall.

IV gamma globulin is given during the acute phase to reduce the risk for coronary artery disease.

Most cases of Kawasaki are seen in children younger than 4.

388) D) Thrombocytopenia is not associated with HSP and anaphylactoid purpura is just another name for HSP.

389) C) This is the classic history and physical findings for **bacterial endocarditis** and also an example of when "reading the question" is critical. You might be tempted to choose D but remember that blood culture, not cardiac echo, confirms the diagnosis of bacterial endocarditis. Remember in clinical practice they may ask you to choose between two studies you would conduct simultaneously; however, on the exam you will need to choose the "definitive test" or the one you would do first.

390) E) Each of the symptoms described are consistent with an initial case of rheumatic fever except answer choice E, which is consistent with a diagnosis of Kawasaki disease.

391) B) High fever, thrombocytosis, sterile pyuria, hydrops of the gallbladder and conjunctivitis can be seen in patients with Kawasaki disease. *Bacterial* meningitis is not associated with Kawasaki. . *Aseptic* meningitis, on the other hand, can be seen in Kawasaki disease.

392) D) Of the all the symptoms listed only palmar erythema is associated with **systemic lupus erythematosus**

393) C) Renal involvement occurs in 75% of patients with lupus usually within 2 years of diagnosis and is a major cause of morbidity and mortality.

394) D Maternal Anti-Ro is the antibody most associated with the development of congenital heart block in newborns.

395) D) The most susceptible racial group for developing lupus are Native Americans, African-Americans are second.

20% of all patients who have lupus are diagnosed before adulthood usually during adolescence rarely in patients younger than 5

After puberty the female male ratio *increases* from 3:1 to 9:1.

Substance Abuse

396) D) **Phentolamine** and **nifedipine** are often used to manage hypertension—*not aggression and agitation*—in an acute overdose of amphetamine and/or methamphetamine. The N-methyl group actually results in an **increase** of the peripheral side effects. The D-form is 5 times more effective than the L-form. Neuroleptics are sometimes used for acute agitation and delirium.

Haldol's onset of action is too slow to have practical application in acute situations, and other forms such as **droperidol** are used.

397) B The most likely explanation in this clinical setting would be glue inhalation. This would not necessarily be deliberate but a distinct possibility in a camp setting. For example this could result if there were an arts and crafts activity using glue containing toluene in a poorly ventilated room.

The key to picking the correct answer is how quickly the symptoms wear off once the child is in the open air.

398) B) The most likely cause of sudden death due to cocaine toxicity would be a cardiac arrhythmia.

399) A   Alprazolam is a benzodiazepine. This could account for the sluggish presentation as well as the equal pupils which are reacting slowly. Marijuana abuse could present similarly but noting the lack of conjunctival injection is the hint that this is not the correct diagnosis.

With heroin abuse you would expect to see constricted pupils.

Amphetamine and phencyclidine (PCP) abuse you would expect to see a more agitated if not paranoid presentation.

400) B)   There is no evidence of acute substance abuse. However there is evidence of hyperpyrexia. Cooling the patient off is critical to reduce the risk of end organ damage. However you want to cool the temperature down to 101.8 but no lower.
Providing a cool glass of water to a patient with blunted mental status would be inappropriate.

Notes

Notes

Notes